Energy Exercises

Easy Exercises for Health and Vitality
Based on Randolph Stone's
Polarity Therapy

Second Edition (Revised)

John Chitty
and
Mary Louise Muller

Illustrations by
Mark Allison

Polarity Press
Boulder, Colorado

ISBN: 978-0-941732-06-2

Library of Congress Control Number: 2017960540

First Edition 1990

Second Edition (Revised) 2018

v.2.0

Disclaimer:

The information in this book is intended for general inquiry and informational purposes only and should not be considered a substitute for medical advice, diagnosis, or treatment. If you think you, or those under your care, are ill or in need of health care, please seek immediate medical attention. Always consult a doctor or other competent licensed clinical professional for specific advice about medical treatments for yourself or those under your care. Any use of, or reliance in any way upon, the information contained in this book is solely at your own risk.

Cover Art: Dani Burke

Energy Exercises

Easy Exercises for Health and Vitality
Based on Randolph Stone's Polarity Therapy

John Chitty and Mary Louise Muller

Art by Mark Allison

Contributing Editors for the 1st Edition

    Mark Allison

    Eileen Bach-y-Rita

    Anna Chitty

    Gail Dennison

    Will Leichnitz

    Kathleen Morrow

    Gary Peterson

    Kathleen Petryshyn

    Sharon Porter

    James Z. Said

    Tom Strathairn

Contributing Editors for the 2nd Edition

    Elizabeth Chitty

Table of Contents

Dedication

In honor of Dr. Randolph Stone,
founder of Polarity Therapy.

"Is it not possible for man to keep well by doing a few simple things daily and by living less strenuously? The answer is yes."

-- Randolph Stone, *Health Building*, p. 101.

"May this work reach the seekers who are looking for a deeper perspective of a common denominator in the healing art, to push it along in keeping with all the other atomic discoveries of today. The health and well-being of the people should not be neglected. It should really be the first concern of the scientists, doctors and educators. Without health and happiness, all our modern conveniences are of little comfort to us."

-- Randolph Stone, *Polarity Therapy Vol. 2*, p. 77.

"Happiness is the consciousness of growth."

-- Alexander Lowen, *Bioenergetics*, p. 33.

Preface

"There must be pioneers for every new idea, or our world
would stagnate and become utterly uninteresting."
-- Randolph Stone, *Polarity Therapy Vol. 2*, p. 103.

This book presents a unique exercise system which is effective for health maintenance and stress relief. The postures are easy to do, requiring little time or effort, and yet they provide great benefits for all ages. These benefits have been proven over many years, with thousands of people, in the practice of Polarity Therapy.

The postures and exercises have many sources. They represent a synthesis of understanding and practices from modern and ancient times, and from West and East. The primary source is the pioneering work of Randolph Stone, founder of Polarity Therapy, to whom this book is respectfully dedicated. His pamphlet "Easy Stretching Postures" was published in 1954 as a way for Westerners to experience some of the benefits of the Eastern health concept of "Energy Balancing."

Randolph Stone, DO, DC, ND
(1890-1981)

Born in Austria, Stone had a medical practice in Chicago for over fifty years. He was an open-minded seeker of knowledge, traveling widely to collect health ideas from around the world, especially India and the Orient. He named his synthesis "Polarity Therapy," a reference to electromagnetic energy dynamics. Stone wrote five books and numerous pamphlets, and taught widely until his retirement in 1974.

1

Polarity Therapy is a uniquely comprehensive model for understanding health. It has a theoretical foundation strong enough to accommodate a wide range of knowledge, old and new, and from many sources.

The deeper origins for these exercises are the ancient traditions of Yoga and Ayurveda in India and Tai Chi and other Martial Arts in East Asia. These venerable systems are not necessarily fully accessible to the busy modern Westerner: the considerable discipline, commitment, study time and supervision associated with these systems make them unavailable for many. The energy exercises presented here extract simple basic movements and postures that anyone can do safely and easily, with little training. Stone's frequent use of the term "Polarity Yoga" indicates the extent of his intention of a linkage between the ancient practices and his modern adaptation.

Stone's work has been supplemented by many people in the field of Polarity Therapy, including Pierre Pannetier (1914-1984), the numerous practitioners of Polarity Therapy throughout the world, and the staff of the Murrieta Foundation. The American Polarity Therapy Association, based in Maryland, is the central voice for Polarity in America today.

A major source of material for this book comes from a branch of the field of Kinesiology. These applications, especially Edu-K (for Educational Kinesiology), have opened dramatic new doors in the therapeutic use of energy concepts. Kinesiology complements Polarity Therapy, while adding significant new material and techniques for energy understanding and balancing.

Similarly, the theories, research and techniques developed out of Craniosacral Therapy are a further advance. These therapies, based on the Osteopathic discovery of subtle rhythmic movements of the cranium and spinal system, echo and confirm central themes in Polarity Therapy, and open broad new possibilities for the field. As an osteopathic physician, Stone was familiar with the basis for these techniques, a personal acquaintance of leading cranial osteopathy practitioners of his day, and author of a significant contribution to the field, *Mysterious Sacrum* (1954). The incorporation of recent advances in Craniosacral Therapy is a natural area of growth for today's Polarity Therapy practitioners.

A fourth major source for this material is the Murrieta Foundation's staff and students. In its different forms, this organization offered Polarity courses between the years 1975 and 1989. It benefited from the involvement of thousands of people at various times, all of whom shared in its vision of making the ideas of Polarity Therapy and natural health better known to the general public. Without this chain of sincere people, this book would not have been created. There are many other influences at work in this book, as represented by the footnotes.[1] To these and others we are grateful for contributing to our growth, and to the expansion of the understanding of energy in the healing arts.

It was Stone's wish that his work not come to an end with his retirement in 1974, and we feel quite certain that he would approve of and participate in new advances. It is in this spirit that this volume is offered, with the hope that it will prove valuable both to those who are familiar with the underlying ideas and their history, and newcomers to the field of wholistic health.

---

[1] We quote widely from many of these sources for several reasons. We hope to give the reader a direct experience of the words of these teachers, and to integrate Polarity Therapy with the larger holistic health movement and with contemporary scientific research findings. We believe that Polarity Therapy as described by Stone is remarkable in its ability to encompass a wide range of subject matter, unifying numerous schools of therapeutic thought in a single comprehensive system. Additionally the wide usage of quotes from related fields is intended to give teachers of Polarity Therapy a good supply of quotable references to use in the presentation of Stone's work.

Notes for the Second Edition

This book was created in 1989, and has been renewed in 2017. Such a long time span involves the progression of discoveries and methods relevant to the topic. We faced a decision about whether to just re-write the whole book to include new information, or to let it stand as a time capsule of its era, with a few additions. We chose the latter, for many reasons, adding just ten new exercises and keeping most of the original text.

Of particular significance for this subject are the greatly expanded (and new since 1990) understandings of neuroscience, including the Autonomic Nervous System and Trauma Resolution. These new developments are game changers for all therapies, and we highly recommend using the new resources that have been developed for the purpose. John Chitty's *Dancing with Yin and Yang* and *Working With Babies* are intended to supply this information area.

Another aspect of this book renewal project was a desire to add a few more drawings. All the original art is by Mark Allison, however for this edition Noah Lohneiss and John Chitty also added graphics. For these new drawings, the initials NL and JC have been added, to distinguish them from the work of the primary artist.

For ease of reading, citations for quotations from Randolph Stone and some others are given at the time of usage, instead of in footnotes.

Introduction: General Principles

This book's exercises are based on the idea of Energy. Practitioners of traditional Eastern medical systems believe that health is a function of a subtle energy which flows in the body. In this book, we describe easy exercises for enhancing, balancing and facilitating this natural energy flow. These are simple postures and movements which give tangible results. Thousands of people have enjoyed these benefits, changing tension and stress to calm, dynamic power.

The idea of energy is ancient, but often new to modern readers. Most of us inherited the world view of Descartes and Newton. Our school training was based on mechanistic, objective, scientific assumptions, while the idea of "Energy" requires a subjective, intuitive attitude.

Here is a selection of comments on the interaction between the old and the new outlooks, from writers in the fields of physics, psychology and medicine.

" ... the classical ideal of an objective description of nature is no longer valid. The Cartesian partition between the I and the world, between the observer and the observed, cannot be made when dealing with atomic matter."
—Fritjof Capra, *The Tao of Physics*, p. 68-69

" ... the question [is] whether an objective scientific view could fully comprehend the functioning... of a human being... Students of personality cannot afford this narrow view."
—Alexander Lowen, *Bioenergetics*, p. 279-280

"Modern medicine is still dominated by the notion that disease is caused by objective agents. A sophisticated analysis shows that this is only partly true."
—Deepak Chopra, *Quantum Healing*, p. 211

To make this new idea easy for newcomers, the start of this book is light on theory and esoteric terminology. We want you to experience the benefits first; if later you want to know why it works, the way is clearly marked. As a start, just enjoy and make good use of the exercises and let them speak for themselves. We believe the words of Stone:

> The Energy Principle is atomic in its concept and is a science of the future... The mechanical approach is totally obsolete in comparison with it... (Stone, *Polarity Therapy Vol. 1*, p. 4.)

When you understand "the Energy Principle," you will understand why the exercises are so effective. In these activities, we work smarter rather than harder.

> This new principle of exercise energy current-release by posture-stretch-relax action is a more natural aid to health than all the forceful muscle straining used in many other methods. (Stone, *Health Building*, p. 100.)

"No force is ever used..." Instead we use an "effortless effort." The effectiveness is due to the use of deeper dimensions of the total person, activating the subtle energy currents, fields and pathways which precede tissues, muscles and organs.

> The postures are given in easy steps, so the process is a natural, progressive approach without force. The postures are designed and used as an easy way of effortless effort, to move the deeper energy currents of the body by a process called "Wu-Wei" in the East. This literally means 'doing by not doing.' Let Mother Nature do it by cooperating with her and resting on her bosom. Thus let the Universal Currents take over the job. It is literally riding the River of life's energy waves and tuning into them. (Stone, *Health Building*. p. 105.)

The basic pulse of life builds and animates all the systems, functions and tissues. These exercises are designed to affect the subtle core energy, and thereby create improvement all the way "downstream" in the denser systems, functions and tissues. Energy exercises affect the entire body through the interrelationship of all systems.

Energy flow feels good! People describe it as warmth, tingling, buzzing or vibration. Stress is reduced and the mind relaxes.

Benefits that you may experience include release of physical or emotional tension, weight loss, relief from pain, broadening of mental perspective, elimination of waste solids, liquids, and gases, intake of new oxygen, restructuring of posture, improved digestion and blood circulation, enhancement of job or athletic performance, and more. Because the system is based on the whole person, benefits arise on levels and in areas which may have seemed unrelated. "Touch one strand and the whole web trembles."[2] Energy is the common thread uniting every aspect of our lives.

Energy: More Than Just Exercise

Energy is affected by one's entire lifestyle. The whole Polarity Therapy system incorporates diet, exercise, bodywork, health information, resolution of emotional issues and realistic thinking. We believe in working with the whole person. Therefore these exercises are just one part of a whole way of life.

Stone compared the body to a house with plumbing, heat, lighting and drainage. This "house" has three levels (mental, emotional and physical) and five phases (space, gas, heat, liquids, solids). An effective health system must incorporate and address the issues of all parts of the whole.

---

[2] Chopra, Deepak. *Quantum Healing: Exploring the Frontiers of Mind-Body Medicine.* Random House, 1989.

It is up to the tenant (the consciousness, soul, or spirit) to keep the house (mind, feelings, body) in good condition, and different tools and specialties are used for different parts of the house. Energy Exercises is one major tool, but the others are also very significant.

> Ultimately it is up to each individual to work toward a continual state of balance; harmonizing of structural, chemical, emotional, spiritual and environmental factors into a lifestyle which enhances health.[3]

---

[3] Thie, John. *Touch for Health.* p. 112.

Part One

A Quick Introductory Tour
of Energy Exercises and Theories

"Energy is the real substance
behind the appearance of matter and form."
(Stone, *Polarity Therapy Vol. 2*, Book 6, p. 4)

A typical beginning routine for energy exercises might include an introduction to the idea of energy, Scissors Kicks, Foot Reflexology, the Pyramid, the Squat, and a closing Light Rocking Perineal. This sequence engages and energizes the major current pathways in the body, and provides a tour of key landmarks in Stone's energy exercise system.

For the introduction to theory, a simple question is asked. Of what are we made? High school science told us the answer is atoms, the primary building blocks of all matter. But the words "building blocks" and "matter," which sound so concrete, can be deceptive.

> Far from being the hard and solid particles they were believed to be since antiquity, the atoms turned out to consist of vast regions of space... It is not easy to get a feeling for the... magnitude of atoms... In order to visualize this diminutive size, imagine an orange blown up to the size of the Earth. The atoms of the orange will then have the size of cherries.... In our picture of cherry-sized

atoms, the nucleus of an atom will be so small that we will not be able to see it... To see the nucleus, we would have to blow up the size of the atom (the cherry) to the size of the biggest dome in the world, the dome of St. Peter's in Rome (138 feet across)... In an atom of that size, the nucleus would have the size of a grain of salt! A grain of salt in the middle of the vast dome of St. Peter's, and specks of dust whirling around it in the vast space of the dome - this is how we can picture the nucleus and electrons of an atom.[4]

With this image in mind, the seeming solidity of the body is less definite. It is a small step further to envision the body as a whirling combination of these spacious "events" called atoms. The most "real" part of the system is not the grains and specks of dust, but rather the awesome force of attraction and repulsion which keeps them in place in extremely complex functions. "Energy," the potential or actual expression of this force, is the primary "glue" of the universe.

Energy is always there, whether we are aware of it or not. Usually we are not, but we can actually feel energy. Place the hands together and rub them briskly.[5] Continue with firm pressure back and forth for at least a minute, or until the arms are tired, whichever comes first. Now, take a deep breath in through the nose and blow it out fully, stopping the hand-rubbing and partially closing the eyes when exhalation is complete. Place the hands close together, not quite touching. Notice sensations in the palms. There will be a warm tingling, from the stimulation of sensory nerves of the palms.

---

[4] Capra, Fritjof. *The Tao of Physics*. p. 65-66. Similarly: "When you get to the level of atoms, the landscape is not one of solid objects moving around each other like a dance, following predictable steps. Subatomic particles are separated by huge gaps, making every atom more than 99.999% empty space." –Chopra, *Quantum Healing*, p. 96.

[5] Gordon, Richard. *Your Healing Hands*. p. 20.

But there is another sensation here also. Experiment with moving the hands further apart, then closer together, then slightly up and down across each other. That light sensation, which rises and ebbs as the hands move closer and further, and feels like corduroy ridges as the fingers pass each other, is energy![6]

Feeling energy is the first step toward appreciating what energy exercises can offer. Learning increased sensitivity is a theme in Energy Exercise classes: when you're sensitive, energy in the hands can be felt without rubbing. Most people have suffered a gradual loss of awareness of their feelings and their bodies. We accumulate our tensions gradually so we don't notice the difference from day to day. We could add one small pebble each day to our load (in the form of a frustrating experience or unresolved conflict) and end up years later under a crushing burden which we never really perceive.

---

[6] Alexander Lowen uses a different hand position to get the effect all the way into the arms. Place the fingers together, in a "praying" pose. Then turn the hands (heels and palms always continuing to touch), so that the fingers point at the chest. This hyperextends the fingers. Hold this position for at least a minute, or as long as you can. Then lightly rest, eyes closed, knees bent, arms hanging loosely. That tingling feeling is also energy! (Lowen, *Bioenergetics,* p. 63).

It is... true that most people are unaware of the bodily handicaps under which they labor - they have become second nature.[7]

This is especially true if we habitually de-sensitize ourselves with painkillers, drugs, alcohol, coffee and other stimulants or depressants. Our everyday state may be tension, which feels "normal" to us. Unfortunately as we get more tense we also become more numb. We value sensitivity less, and become less likely to know what "good" really feels like.

Energy is flowing through the body in specific pathways, like roads carrying traffic through a city. Our goal is smooth traffic flow throughout the system. Unfortunately, there are always interruptions: accidents, flat tires, bad weather and rush hour congestion reduce or slow the flow of traffic. Lack of love, stressful living, bad food and lack of movement have a similar effect in the body: slowing energy flow.

We experience energy blockage as pain and disease. These blockages follow a certain sequence, from subtle to dense manifestation:[8] thoughts affect feelings which affect the physical body. Inefficient or negative attitudes, unrealistic expectations or traumas generate emotionally-charged destructive habits or painful, unresolved, repressed feelings, which lead to physical problems.

Starter Set of Energy Exercises

Our next activity will start to open traffic up and add to our experience of energy. Move down to the floor, on the stomach, head resting on hands. Lift the feet so that the lower leg is perpendicular to the floor. Start the "Scissors Kick" by gently rocking the feet out, then in, back and forth like windshield wipers. The easy, rhythmic movement emphasizes the

---

[7] Lowen, Alexander. *Bioenergetics.* p. 63.

[8] This sequence, "the path to illness," is described by many teachers. For examples, see Franklyn Sills, *The Polarity Process*, p. 85, and Tony Robbins, *Unlimited Power.* p. 40.

Scissors Kick

Pyramid

Foot Reflexology

Quick Tour

An Introduction to Energy Exercises

*Remember to pause and notice the effects
after each exercise!*

outward kick. Continue for a few minutes, rocking the legs
back and forth, alternating either foot crossing on top. Then
roll over and rest, arms either flat to the sides or right hand
on the belly and left hand on the forehead. Feel for the tin-

gling, or wavelike movement across the body. That's energy again, and traffic is starting to move.

Next, roll to the side to a sitting position for a foot reflexology massage. With one leg drawn up, press and stretch the foot in every part and direction. Give each toe a pull. With the toes flexed, press deeply with the thumb on all parts of the sole of the foot. Find the tender areas: these are reflexes to places where the traffic is blocked elsewhere. As you read this book, you will learn what these areas mean. Hold the most tender spot until the tension eases. Use the thumb and fingers of the other hand to grasp and press the Achilles tendon and calves. A good foot massage in the evening is effective first aid for tension accumulated during the day.

After a short rest, stand up for the "Pyramid." Open the stance so that the feet are directly below the knees. The feet should be parallel to the thighs. Lean forward and place the hands just above the knees. Now transfer the weight from the legs and hips to the shoulders and arms. The arms should be straight, the back straight, and the neck relaxed and somewhat retracted into the shoulders, like a turtle. Keep moving slightly from side to side with full breathing, concentrating on the exhalation. Feel the arms pressing the knees wider, the suspension of the lower back, and the energizing of the shoulder blades. After a few moments, before it starts to be a strain, move up to a standing position. Take another moment of rest, breathing normally, eyes partly closed, knees slightly bent.

Next, lift the hands, arms outstretched in front, and cautiously do some light knee bends. Move up and down, each time a little lower, and see how far down you can go. If it's hard to get down to the haunches, put something (a board or a book) under the heels; if balance is a problem, find something to hold for steadiness. Shift slightly from side to side to add to the movement. When ready, stay in the down position, armpits near the knees, resting in the "Squat." Rock slightly,

Squat

Light Rocking Perineal

back and forth and side to side, for as long as comfortably possible. Then put the hands on the floor in front and slowly come back to standing. Finish with a few moments of silent rest, knees lightly bent, eyes partly closed.

Now move back to the floor. To finish, lie back down, on the left side. Curl up partially, with knees up a little. Place the left hand across the chest and up to the right neck/shoulder junction, and the right hand on the right hip. This is the "Light Rocking Perineal." Rock very slightly, using the balance of the body so that little effort is needed. After a few moments of rocking, rest quietly with eyes closed. If you like, roll over to your back for further rest. Then, rise back to standing and "take inventory" of the whole system. Attempt to compare the "flow of traffic" now to the flow at the beginning. You'll find a feeling of ease and relaxation, of vitality and calm power. Welcome to the wonderful world of Energy Exercises!

Now that we have an idea of energy and what it feels like, let's discuss the basic details of how it works. This is the topic of "Energy Anatomy."

3 Principles & 5 Elements

The study of anatomy takes on a new meaning in the energetic approach to health. Instead of tissues, muscles, bones and organs, the "energy anatomy" describes pathways, vibratory frequencies and energy functions.

Combining Eastern health theory with his practical experience, Stone gave thorough descriptions of a "Wireless Anatomy," or the movement of energy through the body. He offered two basic considerations for the mapping of pathways, each with numerous supporting details and features. These two levels of differentiation are called "Energy Principles" and "Energy Elements." The Three Principles and Five Elements are the main concepts in understanding energy anatomy and the theory of energy.

The Three Principles

The Three Principles describe the way energy moves. It pulses out, pulses in, and rests/reverses, in a constant cycle. In the body, energy moves out to the extremities and back to the core in rhythmic pulsations. Blood, breath, nerves: all systems follow this basic pattern of going out, coming back, and stillness. Many names have been given to these. The best known are from China: "Yang" for going out, "Yin" for coming back, and Neutral for the middle transition. In the Vedic

> **Comments on the Three Principles pulsation:**
> "We are a sea of liquids making a structure and shape... a pattern of pulsation leading to certain patterns of experienced life, feeling and thinking both within ourselves and with others... One of the fundamental elements seen in living material is its pulsatory organization, its ability to expand and contract, to lengthen and shorten, to swell and shrink... [Man's] pattern of expansion and contraction organizes basic cognition and perception- empty/full; slow/fast; expand/withdraw; engulf/disgorge. All feeling and thinking is based on this pumping action... Expansion and contraction are the essential pumps of existence."
> -- Stanley Keleman, *Emotional Anatomy*, p. 57, 62
>
> "Modern physics has shown that the rhythm of creation and destruction is not only manifest in the turn of the seasons and in the birth and death of all living creatures but is also the very essence of inorganic matter... the dance of creation and destruction is the basis of the very existence of matter... Modern physics has thus revealed that every sub-atomic particle not only performs an energy dance, but also is an energy dance; a pulsating process of creation and destruction."
> -- Fritjof Capra, *The Tao of Physics*, p. 244.
>
> "This dance of attraction and repulsion between charged particles is called the electromagnetic force. It enables atoms to join together to form molecules and it keeps negatively charged electrons in orbit around positively charged nuclei. At the atomic and molecular level it is the fundamental glue of the universe."
> -- Gary Zukav, *The Dancing Wu Li Masters*, p. 206

tradition from India, the terms are "Rajas" for going out, "Tamas" for coming back and "Satva" for neutral stillness.

The Five Elements

Phenomena appear in stages of increasing density, from light and subtle to heavy and dense. These layers or phases are space, gas, heat, liquid, and solid.

In Polarity Therapy they are called Ether (space), Air (gas), Fire (heat), Water (liquid) and Earth (solid). In the body, five centers called Chakras transform energy, adjusting its density and speed as it moves up and down the body to accomplish different functions.

How Energy Exercises Work

These exercises open energy pathways. Energy blockages, the result of trauma and tension, are cleared out by the combination of methods used in this system. The goal is to optimize the Three Principles and Five Elements so that there is an ease and balance of expansion and contraction in all fields of action, from subtle to dense. Balanced energy flows freely on physical, emotional and mental levels. Energy movement, feeling well and health improvement are directly linked: these exercises can lead to all three, often in a way that can be felt immediately.

The energy that forms and operates the body has a great inner intelligence. It fights germs, heals bumps and bruises, processes emotional experiences and thinks of solutions to complex problems, all far better than could ever be done from outside. In doing energy exercises, learn to tune in to this innate intelligence and assist it in its natural healing work. Therefore these exercises should be done mindfully. Be sensitive to your body's natural biofeedback, and let it guide your choices. The body is a natural self-correcting system; these exercises enhance that self-healing power.

How To Choose Effective Exercises with the Principles and Elements

The Three Principles have basic qualities which are reflected in three types of movement: active for Yang, peaceful for Neutral, and changing for Yin. Intuition can tell when to employ exercises in each category (exercises are categorized by Principles at the end of the book). Perhaps you need to calm down and re-center yourself; the quiet stilling postures of the Neutral Principle would be appropriate. Perhaps you feel a need for greater action and self-expression: for this, use exercises that activate the Yang Principle. When you feel heavy and sluggish, exercises of the Yin Principle will promote a change.

To use the Five Elements to plan exercises, consider their main location and secondary connections as shown below. If you have tension or pain in one or the areas listed in the second column, Energy Exercises based on that element are recommended (exercises are indexed by element at the end of the book). If emotional stress is causing a problem, find the closest approximate term for the feeling in the far right column, and use exercises relating to that element.

Five Elements: Locations, Related Areas and Emotional Qualities					
Element	Main Location	Superior Pole	Neutral Pole	Inferior Pole	Emotional Qualities
Ether	Throat				Self-Esteem, Expression, Grief
Air	Chest	Shoulders	Kidneys	Ankles	Desire, Hope
Fire	Solar Plexus	Head	Solar Plexus	Thighs	Anger, Will Power
Water	Abdomen, Pelvis	Breast	Genitals	Feet	Attachment, Discipline
Earth	Coccyx, Perineum	Neck	Bowels	Knees	Fear, Courage

This approach can be simple or very sophisticated. An example of a simple use would be using Fire Element exercises when anger is being experienced: this vents the pent-up energy in that center and gives relief. As a more complex example, an Earth Element exercise could be beneficial for a person with chronic Air stress in the chest or problems with excessive desires: it would give an earthy grounding of practicality to balance the lofty ambitions. Thus energy exercises become a form of energy balancing, a self-given and self-regulated way to create and maintain inner harmony. These have been proven effective at both beginning and advanced levels.

Get to know the various exercises from both an inner, intuitive sense and an outer, intellectual knowledge of their benefits. You will then be able to use them as your own form of self-help and growth. Many students have said they feel newly empowered in self-care through these exercises, enabling them to work with issues of many kinds, from headaches and indigestion to emotional processing.

Listen to Yourself First

The highest authority on what is going on in your body is you. Others may have knowledge of anatomy or exercise physiology or general rules that work for most people, but your perspective is unique.

Get to know your body and listen to its limitations as well as its needs. Health comes from within. In Energy Exercises, we work with the body, not on it.

Be especially sensitive to pain. Pain can mean several things: that energy is blocked, that the exercise is being done improperly, that you are not ready for it, or that it is just not a good exercise for you. Furthermore, there are "good" pains, like a deep massage, and "bad" pains, indicating undue stress. You are the judge: your body knows the difference and will tell you if you listen.

Ancient Symbols of Energy Anatomy

In developing Polarity Therapy, Stone drew information from the world's great cultures and religions. His books refer to a wide variety of sources, old and new and from East and West.

He was fascinated by ancient symbols. "All these cryptic designs bear a hidden message to thinkers. By knowing them, man can gain intelligent direction and knowledge…" (Stone, *Polarity Therapy Vol 1*, p. 33.)

The Caduceus, an Egyptian and Greek symbol also known as the Staff of Hermes or Staff of Life, attracted Stone's attention. In Roman mythology, the Caduceus was the magic wand of Mercury (called Hermes by the Greeks), son of Jupiter and messenger of the Gods. A gift from Apollo, the Caduceus was used to guide souls in their travels after death. Today, a modified Caduceus serves as the symbol for the medical profession.

Stone explains:

MAN KNOW THYSELF is the admonition contained in the symbolism of the Staff of Hermes.

"The wings of the Caduceus represent the two hemispheres of the brain. The knob in the center is the pineal body. The upright staff is the path of the finer energy of the brain and the spinal chord below it..."

The two serpents represent the Mind Principle in its as the vital energy on the right side of the body. It was called Yang by the Chinese... On the left side of the body flows the cooling energy of the Moon essence of nature. It was called Yin by the Chinese...

These two currents cross over in each oval cavity [five in number] and change their polarity. Thus they flow

The Caduceus
Ancient Symbol of Energy in the Body

Three Principles:
The snakes represent the Yin and Yang currents, and the staff represents the neutral current. The globe at the top represents the brain, and the wings represent consciousness.

Five Elements:
The five junctions and oval cavities manage specific functions in the body.

in and out of each other constantly and produce alternating currents in their action...

The knowledge of these currents [the Three Principles], and the relationship of these ovals [the Five Elements]... was the understanding of the physicians of old. It is concealed and revealed in this symbol of the Caduceus. (Stone, *Polarity Therapy Vol. 1*, p. 33.)

The Tao

At least as old as the Caduceus, the east Asian symbol of Yin and Yang also depicts the Three Principles concept. Light and dark represent a dynamic cycle of opposites that are constantly becoming each other. The third neutral principle is expressed by the balance of the two polarities.

Babbitt's Atom

Drawing from another more modern resource, Stone used Dr. Edwin Babbitt's design to illustrate the essential form of energy fields.[9] Midlines, spirals and pulsatory action are the "laws of form." In humans, the midline is the spine, spirals are visible in the fingerprints and the crown of the head, and pulsations such as the heart's rhythm are a key to all function. Other structures such as the rib cage, sea shells, pine cones and the DNA double helix have similar shapes.

---

[9] Babbitt, Edwin. *Principles of Light and Color.* First published in 1873, reprinted in 1993 by Sun Publishing.

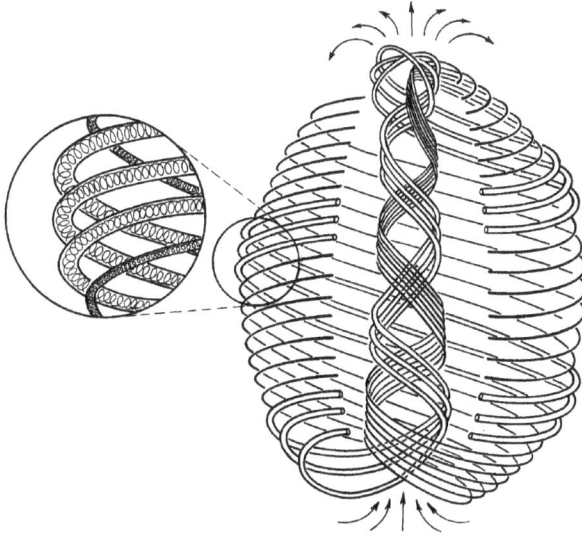

If we could see the electromagnetic field of the human body, it would look something like this.

Atomic Science

Stone observed in 1948 that the Three Principles idea was reflected in then-new discoveries of the atom.

> This triune arrangement is the basis of all matter in motion and expression, even as the atom is the unit of it. (Stone, *Polarity Therapy Vol. 1, I Book 3*, p. 8.)

The same attraction-repulsion bonding that holds an atom together can be seen in many other natural phenomena, such as molecular bonding and magnetism. Stone concluded that the familiar shapes of nature represent fundamental aspects of reality, leading to a guiding cosmology for his health care system.

This Book's Logo

The Three Principles and Five Elements are also represented in this book's decor: the principles are the mountains, while the elements are the petals and center of the central lotus design.

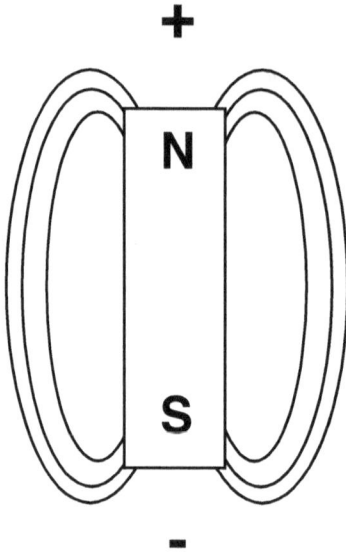

The shape displayed by iron filings over a bar magnet reveals the basic energetic template for form. All structures have polarized electromagnetic fields, from microscopic to macroscale systems.

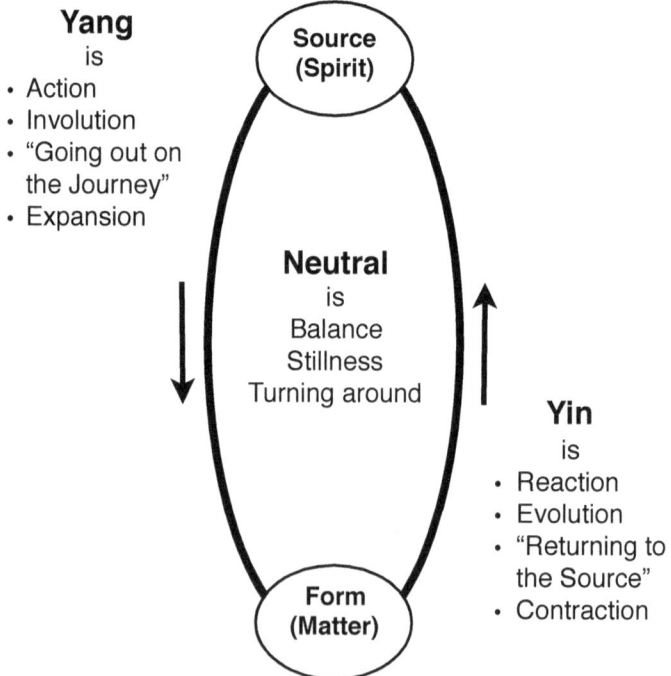

Yang
is
- Action
- Involution
- "Going out on the Journey"
- Expansion

**Source
(Spirit)**

Neutral
is
Balance
Stillness
Turning around

**Form
(Matter)**

Yin
is
- Reaction
- Evolution
- "Returning to the Source"
- Contraction

In numerous diagrams, Stone filled in a complete picture of the energetic substrate of the human form:

CHAKRAS

Where energy is transformed to slower frequencies for performing specific functions.

5. Ether

4. Air

3. Fire

2. Water

1. Earth

This is Stone's illustration for the energy field of the body. The Caduceus in the center creates the Chakras, or energy centers. Radiating out from each Chakra are the spiral circuits of each Element, expressed in the five fingers and toes. All points along lines like these are linked by electromagnetic connections, forming what Stone called "The Wireless Anatomy."

Caduceus
Locating the centers of transformation along the spine.

The Ways Energy Moves
From the core pattern of the Caduceus, energy becomes a radiant pulsing field of spiral-based flow patterns.

Neutral
Side to side
Balance
Satva

Yang
Front-Back
(+) Action
Rajas

Composite
Showing the weaving effect created by the Three Principles.

Yin
Top-Bottom
(-) Reaction
Tamas

Reflexology Zones of the Three Principles

⊕ positive

⓪ neutral

⊖ negative

transverse arch

diaphragm

navel

pelvis

The feet are the negative pole of the brain!

Repeating patterns are the basis for Reflexology. This chart shows Three Principles "zones." The same concept of zones can be used with the Five Elements, as shown on the following page.

"As Above, So Below" is the first statement of the Hermetic Philosophy, an ancient expression of the essential linkage of all levels in any system, supposedly articulated in "The Emerald Tablet of Hermes," ca. 500 BCE or earlier.

Reflexology Zones of the Five Elements

The Five Elements are also expressed in repeating patterns; notice the similarity of shape between areas. The jaw fits into the pelvis, the diaphragm matches lines on the face. **The Ether Element** is in the throat and its reflexes are found in the thumbs and big toes, and also the joints.

Air: Cheeks, Eyebrows, Chest and "pointer" fingers/toes

Fire: Nose, Solar Plexus and middle fingers/toes

Water: Mouth, Pelvis and ring fingers/toes;
Earth: Jaw, Pelvic Floor and little fingers/toes

Eight Methods of Exercise

In Energy Exercises, we use eight techniques:

Lengthening refers to a gentle increase of the length a muscle can have. It can be as simple as reaching out with the arms, or moving the head from side to side. Many of the exercises in this book make use of natural leverage to create lengthening in specific areas of the body. Properly done, lengthening prompts the muscle to reset at a new, longer length.

Lengthening does not mean strain or stretch beyond the limit of range of motion, which tends only to cause reactive tightening afterward. The term lengthening is offered to the exercise world as an alternative to the word "stretch." Stretch suggests a rubber band reaction which snaps back and nullifies the benefit of the exercise.

Pressure refers to direct touch on the body. Pressure can be light, moderate or deep, and it can be moving or still. Pressure has two main uses: for energy balancing (as discussed below) and for tissue release.

Firm pressure can be painful, but pain is not the point. Ideally, firm pressure finds the edge of resistance and does not cause defensive responses. If the pain is an indicator of blocked energy, continued firm contact will facilitate release, not more resistance. Release can be felt in the hands and the body; tingling, pulsation and warmth replace the pain.

For tissue release, pressure can be used strategically in a number of ways. Within each muscle are mechanisms to monitor the tension which that muscle exerts on tissues and bones. The spindle cell mechanism in the belly of the muscle monitors length. To relax a muscle that is tight, first push into the belly of the muscle above and below its center, then direct the pressure of the fingers toward each other. The muscle gets a message that there is too much contraction and the brain sends a message to lighten up, causing relaxation.

A second mechanism regulating tension is the Golgi apparatus. Muscles are attached to bones by tendons. At the end of the muscle in the tendon area, the Golgi apparatus sends messages to protect the muscles from exerting too much pressure, which could break the bone or tear the tendon. Applying sensitive pressure to the areas where muscles originate or insert in the bone resets the Golgi apparatus and thus relaxes the muscle.

Activation means using a muscle lightly against resistance, followed by release. Muscles work in pairs to exert force across joints creating flexion (shortening across the joint) and extension (lengthening across the joint).

Activation techniques consist of extending a joint as far as is comfortable, then lightly flexing in the opposite direction against resistance with an exhalation. This is repeated: each time the flexing/exhaling is finished, further extension becomes possible, and muscles which were very tight are dramatically lengthened. The body uses force in the flexing direction and as it relaxes from that, further extension happens naturally. Thus lengthening is achieved with less force on the joint that is extending.

Lightness of touch and sensitivity are essential. This is not like isometric resistance used in muscle building, it is a gentle and sensitive way to increase flexibility and range of movement. It is an excellent companion to bodywork, creating relaxation much more efficiently than mechanical stretching.

Breathing refers to conscious inhalation and exhalation, often timed with specific movements, sometimes combined with sound. One group of exercises in this book deals with breathing only. In other exercises breath is coordinated with the exercise. Breathing contributes physical, emotional and esoteric benefits to Energy Exercises. Conscious breathing is so important that some therapies have achieved great success using breath-oriented practices exclusively.

The physical benefits of conscious breathing, especially oxygenation, are well known. Randolph Stone also described a less familiar idea:

> When the breath is used in a posture, it is for a general stretch of the tissues from within, outward, in order to reverse the day-long pressures from without, pushing inward. (Stone, *Health Building*, p. 101.)

A more esoteric dimension of breath is found in the concept of Prana or Life Force. This subtle cosmic energy is considered to be conducted in the air (also, on sunlight and in flowing water). In esoteric philosophy, breathing means absorbing Prana, nourishing the most subtle functions of consciousness and life.

Energy Balancing can mean a number of techniques. "Energy" refers to energy currents and fields in the body, and "balance" describes reducing surplus or increasing deficiency to achieve an equality of force/flow amplitude and a symmetry of distribution.

Energy balancing usually involves the use of hands to contact specific key spots on the body. The hands are like jumper cables for a car battery. Energy flowing between the hands supplements the existing current along particular pathways. The increased circulation has a balancing effect. The pathways may be compared to water streams, which are washed free of sediment by increased flow. Polarity, Reflexology, Shiatsu, Touch for Health, Do-in, Acupressure, Ayurveda and many other health systems employ energy balancing.

"Bodywork" is a generic term that includes energy-balancing contact. More information on the how and why of bodywork is given under "Balancing Touches" (page 131).

Differentiation consists of consciously moving the body in a way that "differentiates" the various parts that are involved in the motion. This approach was developed by Dr. Moshe Feldenkrais. The movement sequences are executed gently and slowly with great mindfulness. Moving slowly while noticing the details, such as the quality and level of comfort, gives the brain the type of sensory/motor stimulation present in the successful learning of motor skills. Under these conditions the brain has the time and freedom to make adjustments and to alter habitual limitations in movement. Slowly, body movements become easy, pain-free and efficient; the mind becomes calm and thinking becomes more clear.

Movement means easy motion, either according to specific instructions or free and without specific form. Movement increases circulation, fires neural circuits and exercises muscles. It can be used to bring life to an area of the body that has become tense and blocked. Stretching, rocking, bending, unbending and rotating are movements used to release and energize.

Sound is an important part of this system and refers to the several ways the voice and other sources are used to create relaxation and energy balancing. As with breathing, sound has many esoteric dimensions and implications. In addition to its use with many exercises, sound has its own section, on page 163.

Part Two:
Exercises
Listed by Body Area

Neck and Shoulders

The neck and shoulders area is the "positive pole" of the torso's electromagnetic field. The neck is the location of the Ether Element center, and the chest is the location of the Air Element center.

The neck is affected by experiences relating to self-expression and making choices. Pride, shame and longing for worldly or spiritual motives manifest here. Sound is an important part of Energy Exercises for the neck area, so the neck will benefit by all postures which employ sound; this includes many of the exercises in this book.

The shoulders are affected by experiences relating to desire, hope and ambition. Tension here comes from "carrying the weight of the world," and from the pressure of unfulfilled wants for ourselves or others.

The interrelationship of body areas is a theme which will be found over and over in this book. Imagine a playground seesaw, with one end directly moving the other. Similarly, the pelvis and shoulders affect each other across the "fulcrum" of the diaphragm.

> The superior acts on the inferior and the inferior supports and reacts on the superior pole. (Stone, *Polarity Therapy Vol. 2*, p. 21.)

Thus the organization of this book by body areas must be approached with a major caution, the understanding that no body area or posture has an isolated existence or effect.

1. Shoulder Reflexes

"A few seconds on the right reflex does wonders."
(Stone, *Polarity Therapy Vol. 2*, p. 85.)

Reflexology means making use of the energy links which exist between seemingly unrelated parts of the body. Beginners are advised just to get started and let the technique speak for itself: reflexology and its benefits are easier to experience than to explain.

For the neck and shoulders, important reflexes are found where the toes join the foot. In classes, we often have participants take a shoulder-lengthening pose such as the Cliffhanger (page 40) or the Pyramid (page 97) for a few seconds first, to gauge the degree of flexibility and to give a standard for comparison.

This is a way to give participants a direct experience of the power of reflexology. Assume one of these poses "cold" (without prior warm-up), do the foot reflexology techniques in the next paragraph, then immediately go back to the test posture. Typically, the Cliffhanger or Pyramid will be difficult before foot reflexology, and noticeably easier after.

Reflexes to the neck are located in the "neck" of each toe, especially the big toe. Massage these areas, feeling for tender spots. When you find areas that are sore, gently push in and hold for a count of at least eight, with full breathing and emphasized exhalation.

Caution
✳

Certain exercises have this mark, indicating that they require special caution. Listen to your body first. All exercises are to be done with care and consciousness. You are the best judge in choosing exercises and doing them in a way that works best for you.

For foot reflexology to benefit the shoulders, flex the foot (toes pulled up as close to the leg as possible), then stretch the toes either up or down, and press the areas at the bases of the toes.

> The main point here is the discovery that the foot must be flexed under a little tension so the areas involved are brought out for all foot therapy applications. (Stone, *Polarity Therapy Vol. 2*, p. 72.)

Be creative: using your feelings and intuition as a guide, stretch and press all around the horizontal zone relating to the Air Element, on top and bottom. This pressure can be quite deep, stimulating with movement, or light. On the top, press around each tendon going to the toes. On the bottom, concentrate on the area around the ball of the foot. Also on the bottom, lift the second toe up and use your thumb to find its tendon underneath. Each toe corresponds to an energy center, and pressure along this tendon affects the chest/

Reflexology: Toes and Neck/Shoulders

Shoulders

Air Element

Ether
Air
Fire
Water
Earth

For the neck, press the base of the toe; for the shoulders, press where the toe joins the foot, and on the second toe generally.

Neck

shoulders area. Follow this tendon down the foot with pressure and movement. Similar tendon pressure is useful for each of the other energy centers: big toe for the neck, second toe for chest, third for solar plexus, fourth for pelvis, and fifth for the pelvic floor.

After pressing on the reflex area, hold the reflex spot on the foot with one hand while the other hand firmly grasps the tissue at the top of the shoulder. Hold this "energy balancing" pose quietly for a minute or so, and observe the effect.

An activation technique can be used with the toe stretch to facilitate release. To do this, take one toe and bend it back to its comfortable limit. Now inhale. Relax. As you exhale, push the toe into the fingers as if unbending it into the resis-

**Foot Reflexology
for the Neck and Shoulders**
"Hand Meets Foot, Shoulders Win"

**Face Reflexology
for the Neck and Shoulders**
"Ridge Meets Bridge"

tance of the fingers. Inhale, relax and with your hand take up any slack, gently bending the toe further back. Repeat as many times as you feel continued easy release.

Toe activation has many uses in bodywork and exercise therapy. Activating the corresponding toe can be valuable as a specific treatment for an energy center. This technique is highly recommended for bodyworkers.

Next is an efficient shoulder reflex technique in which the fingers are intertwined with the toes. Our artist calls this "Hand Meets Foot, Shoulders Win." This will be easy for some, difficult for others, who will have to pull the toes apart one by one to make spaces for the fingers. The fingers should be as close to the base of the toes as possible. Once you have the position, wait for at least one full minute, breathing fully and emphasizing exhalation. Then stretch the toes forward and back and rotate.

A second useful reflex to the junction of the neck and shoulders is where the nose meets the eyebrow line, "where the bridge meets the ridge." The entire eyebrow line is a reflex to the shoulders and may be gently pressed with small circular movements. Concentrate on tender spots just to either side of the nose.

A third reflex, described more fully later because it is commonly used to affect the diaphragm, is the web of the hand, between the thumb and first finger. Firm pressure here is a specific energizer for the throat and neck area.

Benefits
- Release of shoulder and neck tension.
- Increased foot flexibility.
- Good for overall relaxation.

References
Stone, R. *Polarity Therapy Vol. 1*, Book 2, pp. 11, 37, 40, 44, 80.
Stone, R. *Polarity Therapy Vol. 2*, p. 105 ff., pp. 183-184.
Berkson, Devaki. *The Foot Book: Healing the Body through Foot Reflexology*, pp. 46-53.

Gach, Michael. *Acu-Yoga*, p. 136.
Mahoney, Frank. *Hyperton-X*, p. 57

2. Rocking Cliff

This exercise is called the "Rocking Cliff' because it is a warm-up for the more strenuous "Cliffhanger" which follows next in this chapter. Leverage is used to release tension in the shoulders and related areas, and movement is used to influence energy circuits.

Method

The original version of the Rocking Cliff is very simple. Sit comfortably in a chair. With straight arms, support some of the weight of the body by pushing down on the chair and suspending the torso from the shoulders. Now rock back and forth, backward and forward, feeling a gentle movement in the brachial plexus. The shoulder blades start to move and the upper back is relaxed.

Rocking Cliff
Evolutionary (at left) and Involutionary (at right) positions are coordinated with breathing and flexing the brachial plexus.

A second, better-known version has been developed over the years. In this version, the chest is thrust forward and arched back with each rocking movement, as shown in the illustration. Inhale and rock back, rounding the back and feeling a lengthening across the shoulders as you expand the chest with a full breath. Exhale and rock forward, pulling the shoulders back and keeping the chin tucked in.

This version of the posture is valuable for its action on the geometric postures of involution and evolution, curving the torso inward and outward. Inward and outward poses are found in many sources, with many variations: in Hatha Yoga, they are recognizable in several forms, including the Cat, Cow, Bow, Leaf and Cobra postures. Involution and evolution are especially emphasized in Polarity Therapy as an advanced use of the Three Principles idea. The breathing pattern matches the posture's movement, with the Yang inhalation coinciding with the involutionary, inward, rear position, and the Yin exhalation coinciding with the evolutionary, outward, forward position.

Benefits
- Releases tension from the shoulders, neck and upper back.
- Opens breathing: beneficial for people with bronchial and asthmatic conditions.
- Integrates and balances top/bottom (Yin) and front/back (Yang) energy currents.

References
Stone, R. *Health Building,* p. 180. This comes from Sam Busa's "Health Building Yoga," a South African magazine article published in the early 1970s and reprinted in the CRCS edition of *Health Building.*

Berkson, Devaki. *Healing the Body through Foot Reflexology,* pp. 81-83. Berkson presents traditional hatha yoga poses for curving the back outward (the bow), then inward (the leaf) and adds: "This is the most important exercise in this book!" She calls it the "Reflexology Wake Up Exercise."

3. Cliffhanger

The Cliffhanger is one of Stone's best known postures. The use of strategic leverage is the key to this exercise, and sound and breath are emphasized. The shoulder-hip energy link is dramatically used.

The shoulder level base and the hip level base must be engaged simultaneously in the one stretching posture to move the gross energy blocks by means of the subtle energy in the united action on both levels.

The Cliffhanger should be used with caution by beginners. Many people need to use the variations first to avoid over-straining. Instructors are advised to be alert for those who may have difficulty with the Cliffhanger, and to carefully use warm-up exercises, including reflexology and lengthening, to prepare.

Method

For the Cliffhanger, a table or surface is needed, about as high as the thigh or hip. It needs to be quite stable and sturdy: a massage table or an office desk are possibilities. Stand with your sacrum and heels of the hands resting on the edge of the table and your feet shoulder-width or slightly more apart.

Caution
✳
Shoulders

Cliffhanger

If the shoulders feel too stressed, put the feet closer under the torso to partially carry its weight.

Place your hands on the table edge to either side of your body, with the elbows over the wrists. Take a test run by lowering your body. Your back maintains very light contact with the table as you drop down with knees bent as shown in the illustration.

In this lowered position, most of the body weight is on the hands, with the torso "suspended" from the edge of the table. The pelvis should "hang" from the spine: avoid tightened buttocks or stomach muscles. Feel the opening in the arms and chest and experiment with different pelvic and foot positions. Seek a relaxed posture: breathe easily, and let your head rest down. Bring yourself up, using the legs to take the pressure off the arms. The simplest version of the Cliffhanger is just a few repetitions of this up-and-down action.

For a more advanced version, stay in the lower position longer and add conscious breathing. Start with a "cleansing breath." Take a deep breath in through the nose, and give a full, complete exhalation through the mouth. Then inhale again, and as you exhale with a deep "a-a-a-h-h" sound, glide your back down the table edge. Lower the body down until you feel resistance in the shoulders.

Support your body weight with your legs only as much as necessary to avoid straining (having the feet close in gives more support, having the feet further out gives more stretch). If your shoulders are loose, let the body's entire weight hang on the arms. If they are tight, use the legs for partial support.

Push the sound out with the diaphragm until all air is out. Come up, wait a moment, stand away from the table, then inhale. Remain in a relaxed standing pose for at least 30 seconds, with a sensitive attitude, to experience the results.

If this is easy for you, you are ready to do a series of releases; if this is not easy, go back to reflexology for the shoulders. Inhale, and as you exhale with an "aah" sound, go down again to the point of resistance. Stay there after exhaling (blowing all the air out through the mouth) fully and then inhale again, allowing the internal pressure of the full breath to press in to areas of tension in the chest and shoulders. Then exhale and relax down even further. On the next inhale, either come up or continue with one or two more inhale-exhale cycles. As you exhale you may push the shoulder blades together in the back to increase the release. Experiment with slowly moving the hips, legs, head and elbows in this fully lowered position.

When you are finished with the last exhale, make sure to blow all the air out and then stand up with lungs empty. This is difficult to do since we tend to want to fill up again right away. Allow yourself to stay empty for a moment. Stand empty and blow out any more air that might be left. By making the emptiness as complete as possible, we create more potential for intake of fresh air. Then, take a breath through the nose. Feel how full, satisfying and refreshing that first breath is. Notice any new sensation.

A full series for an advanced session can be three or more up-and-down cycles, with three or more "aah" breaths each.

Variations

For a less difficult Cliffhanger, use a ledge that is close to the floor. The floor supports the body weight in the down position, instead of having all the weight carried by the shoulders. A low couch or coffee table can work well. In a chair, the chair back can be used as the ledge. This way you can enjoy the opening of the chest and shoulders without the suspension. In a "seated" position with the arms reaching up and back as shown in the illustration, do the same inhale and "aah" exhale sequence. Experiment with rotating the shoulder blades toward each other, or up and down. Remember to keep the head down and neck relaxed, and to take a moment afterward to experience the results.

An easier possibility is illustrated on page 179 of *Health Building*; this is a cross between the Cliffhanger and the

Pyramid. An armchair is used for support in this variation. From a seated position, place the arms on the side armrests. Lift the body by pressing down with the arms, and follow the same breathing sequence described above.

Benefits
- Release of tension in the chest, neck, shoulders, diaphragm and pelvic areas.
- Opens the brachial plexus, which Stone called "the Governor of the Breath," (Stone, *Polarity Therapy Vol. 1*, Book 3 Chart 62.) regulating whether the breath is deep and full or just enough to maintain life.
- Increases the capacity to breathe deeply, feel and give and take fully with the world around us. This has significant emotional and mental implications.
- Opens the chest for breathing and inspiration. Ventilates unused lung areas, increasing elimination of carbon dioxide and intake of oxygen.
- Opens rounded shoulders or a concave chest.
- Unbinds over-developed, over-muscular brachial plexus areas.
- Frees the shoulder blades from being overly bound to the ribs. "The sicker the patient is, the tighter the shoulder blades are on the ribs." (Stone, *Polarity Therapy Vol. 1*, Book 3, p. 18.)
- Preventative for heart conditions; opens heart area.
- Reflexology effects include hyperextension of wrist (pelvic reflex, see Zones chart, p. 27).

References
Stone, R. *Health Building*, pp. 170, 172-173, 180.
Stone, R. *Polarity Therapy Vol. 1*, Book 3, pp. 18-19.
Seidman, Maruti. *Polarity Therapy*, p. 138.
Seigel, Alan. *Polarity Therapy*, p. 78.
Francis, John. *Polarity Self-Help Exercises*, pp. 35-36.
Lowen, Alexander. *The Way to Vibrant Health*, p. 95.

4. Shoulder Shrug Neck Roll

This exercise uses dynamic shoulder/neck action to release hard-to-get areas. It is one of those movements that people do spontaneously for stress relief, without knowing why it works. Baseball players do a version of this just before batting, and golfers just before an important shot.

Method

Stand or sit in a relaxed position. For part one, shrug the shoulders up, bringing them toward the neck area, so the neck seems to disappear and you look a bit like a penguin.

Shoulder Shrug
*Upward Arches
and Downward Arcs*

Hold this shrug and lift your chin up. Now begin to make slow "upward arches," arcing the chin left and then right. Inhale one direction, exhale the other. Do this four or five times, or until the release feels complete, and then return to the middle position. Keep the shoulders up and now bring the chin down.

Next, with the chin down, begin to make a similar movement in a downward direction. Arc the chin left and then right. Inhale one direction and exhale the other. When done, return to the middle position and allow your shoulders to relax down. Give the arms a shake-out, shrug the shoulders once or twice, and check how they feel. Also, check how your neck feels when you rotate it.

For part two, repeat this same process with the shoulders down. Pretend you are carrying big pails of water which are weighing your arms and shoulders down. Keep the shoulders down and repeat the same movements, first "upward arcs" upward, then "downward arcs" downward. Again shake-out, shrug the shoulders, and check the range of motion in the shoulders and neck.

Variations

Place your finger on your nose to mark center position. Now while keeping your finger still, and your nose touching the finger, slowly rotate the chin left and then right while keeping the shoulders pulled down. The head movement "hinges" on the unmoving finger. Hold and feel for the release and lengthening of neck and shoulder muscles.

Benefits
- Release of shoulder and neck tension.
- Lengthening of muscles, helping the neck area to self-correct and adjust itself.

References
Dennison, Paul and Gail. *Brain Gym*, p. 9-10.

5. Neck & Shoulder Tapping

Hamilton and Elizabeth Barhydt's exercise system is based on Chinese acupuncture and Kinesiology. For a discussion of the link between Polarity Therapy (primarily from India) and acupuncture (from China), see page 253. The tapping technique is used in many other energy balancing techniques, and in traditional massage. Tapping is found in the Thymus Thump and Fountain of Love (pages 162 and 160), and it can be done anywhere on the body for stimulating benefit.

Method

For shoulders, tap with the fingertips in the hollow of the shoulder. For the neck, tap an acupressure point in the stomach midway between the navel and the xiphoid process (the cartilage tip at the bottom of the sternum). These points are on the appropriate acupuncture meridians. When finished, take a quiet moment to feel the results on neck and shoulder areas.

Benefits

• Stimulates energy flow in reflex areas, assisting relaxation of muscles.

Reference

Barhydts, Harrison and Elizabeth. *Self-Help for Stress and Pain*, p. 32.

6. The Owl

This exercise releases the shoulder and neck area, especially the trapezius and brachial plexus.

Method

Grasp the fleshy area on the top of your shoulder and maintain a firm yet sensitive grip. Inhale and turn your head toward that shoulder until you can look back over it. Exhale and turn your head toward the other shoulder. Repeat this several times and then return the head to the middle. Now inhale and lift your chin up. Exhale and lower the chin to-ward your chest. After doing this several times, return the head to the middle, relax your grip and feel the change in the shoulder area. Then, repeat the sequence with the other shoulder.

Variations

Grasp the shoulder and again rotate the head toward the shoulder you are gripping. Continuing this firm grasp, lift the arm out on that side with the thumb up and move the arm back behind you. Then turn the head back the other way, while keeping the arm back. As you again turn toward the gripped shoulder allow your arm to float back further if it can. Repeat this several times and then do the other shoulder and arm.

Stone presents a related treatment which affects the neck a little higher in the same general area. Instead of reaching across to hold the shoulder, reach up and over the head. For most people, the fingertips will reach down to the top or middle of the neck. Give a light pull once or twice, breathing deeply with an emphasis on the exhalation.

The Owl

A combination of this variation with an activation technique is very good for shoulder relaxation. Reach the right hand across the head, holding above the ear on the left side. Put the left hand on the left shoulder, middle and index fingers pressing into the spot where neck and shoulder meet.

Lengthen the head to the right as you inhale, then activate by pressing the head into the right hand, toward the left side as you exhale. Inhale and relax, allowing the head and neck to lengthen further toward the right. Repeat this three times, then do the other side. This can be an excellent break from concentrated office or computer work.

Benefits
- Release of shoulder and neck tension. The Owl is especially good during concentrated reading, computer work, telephoning or other desk work.
- Encourages full breathing.

References
Dennison, Paul and Gail. *Brain Gym*, p. 17.
Stone, R. *Health Building*, p. 147.
Stokes, Gordon and Whiteside, Daniel. *One Brain*, p. 30.

7. Vagus Stimulation

The Vagus Nerve (Cranial Nerve X) runs from the brainstem through the neck to innervate the viscera. The Vagus is important in a host of parasympathetic autonomic functions, such as baseline metabolism, digestion, circulation and elimination. But it also is a portal into the Autonomic Nervous System (ANS) generally. Since the ANS is arguably the foundation of health, Vagus nerve stimulation can be a way to support the entire system. Vagus nerve effects may be a subtle reason that neck rubs feel so good and create such a warm

Vagus
Nerve
Access
at the →
neck

JC

48

glow throughout the body.

The significance of the Vagus nerve is confirmed by the effectiveness of Vagus nerve pacemaker devices, which are used for a host of conditions including depression and seizures. Some of the puzzling effects of whiplash injuries, such as digestive problems, sleep disorders and psychological complications, may be Vagus nerve effects.

In addition, the Vagus nerve is thought to be a factor in infant colic, as the nerve is vulnerable to bruising pressure at the jugular foramena (in the suture between the occiput and temporal bones) during birthing. The baby's head passes first across the mother's sacral promontory and then her pubic bone; these solid contacts can press on the cranial bones and cause them to bump the Vagus as it passes from inside the cranium to begin its descent through the neck.

Method

To stimulate the Vagus nerve, visualize its pathway through the neck. It lies under the muscles directly below the ear. Use a firm circular stroking motion on both sides, deeply massaging the tissues for three or four minutes. Imagine that the Vagus is being squeezed and released by the fingertip

Vagus Nerve Stimulation
The sides of the neck and specific points on the ear have been used for vagus stimulation with medical devices, and the benefits are also available through touch.

NL

49

pressure. Complete the experience by resting quietly for an equal amount of time that was spent massaging, imagining the pathway as being fully functional.

Benefits

• Soothing for the whole Autonomic Nervous System including its stress responses and the normal functioning that governs the digestive and circulatory systems.

References

Stone, R. *Polarity Therapy Vol. 1*, Book 3, Chart 23.
Stone, R. *Polarity Therapy Vol. 2*, Book 6, Chart 20, Fig. 2.
Huang, F. et al. "Vagus Stimulation" in *Complementary & Alternative Medicine 2014*, reported in *Science News* Oct. 28, 2015.

Related Exercises

Rocking V (p. 54)
Tummy Rock (p. 136)

8. Arm Activation

This activity is an excellent release for the arm muscles that originate in the chest and shoulders. Releasing these muscles relaxes neck and shoulder tension and energizes the the chest and back. It also enhances communication between the brain and hands.

Method

Start with the right arm, by raising it straight up. Wrap the left hand around it, as shown in the illustration. The left hand creates an isometric resistance with the right arm, pushing against it in an activation movement. Activate the arm in four different directions: to the side, back, toward the head, and forward. For each direction, the left hand will be moved and relocated so that it provides resistance for each direction.

First, place the left hand so it wraps around the outside of the right arm. Inhale and as you exhale through pursed lips, push the right arm out using approximately 25% of your full muscle strength. As with most activation techniques, the arm will not really move: the two arms counterbalance each other. As you inhale, relax and allow the arm to lengthen. You may repeat this several times, do the other arm, or move to the next hand position.

In step two, place the left hand so it creates a flat surface behind the right arm. Now activate, pushing back on the exhale and relaxing/lengthening on the inhale.

For step three, place the left hand so it pushes the right arm away from the head. Activate by pushing the arm in on the exhale and relaxing and lengthening on the inhale.

For step four, place the left hand in front of the right arm, using either the palm or back of the hand, whichever is easier. Activate by pushing forward on the exhale and releasing-lengthening on the inhale. Once you are familiar with this exercise, you can do the complete series easily and quickly by activating on the exhale and moving to a new hand position as you lengthen and relax on the inhale.

Notice that pressing forward and inward affects the chest muscles, while pressing back and outward uses the back muscles.

Arm Activation
Use isometric resistance to release arm and shoulder muscles.

Repeat the whole sequence for the opposite side.

Variations

This activation of the arm can be used in any direction, any part of the arm (upper or lower), and in any posture. Experiment with different muscles to experience its value.

Activation for the neck and head is similar to arm activation, an isometric release for the neck. It can be done in any direction: experiment to feel what is best for you. A detailed variation is given with the Owl posture on the preceding pages.

The technique is familiar: place one hand against the head, and press against it with 25% of neck strength as you exhale through pursed lips. Release pressure as you inhale, and allow the neck to lengthen before repeating or going to a new position. Do one side, then the other, then front and back.

For bodyworkers, massage therapists and physical therapists, we recommend activation techniques such as these for any area of the body as a safer, easier alternative to conventional mechanical stretching. With creativity, most muscles can be opened and relaxed through activation, including such important, but sometimes difficult, muscles as the hamstring.

Benefits
• Good for desk workers who need an open flexible link between the brain and the hands, it opens the energy links and pathways across the shoulders.

References
Dennison, Paul and Gail. *Brain Gym*, p. 18.

9. Head Lift

Neck muscles are often tense and contracted. This postural exercise is a gentle reminder to elevate the head and hold the shoulders back. It is a good discipline to add to walking. The erect posture which this develops reminds us of the dignified upright pose seen in Egyptian art, with the head held high and the back straight.

Method

Imagine having a string attached to the back of your head. As you stand or walk, lift the head up from the back as if pulled by the string from above, tucking the chin down in front slightly. Drop the shoulders allowing the neck to hang from the head. You may be able to feel relaxation as far down as the upper back. The shoulders, diaphragm and pelvis are all affected by this "re-structuring" posture.

10. Rocking V

Stone called this "Polarity Exercise for the Release of the Brachial Plexus and Neck Tension." It has also been called the Spinal Roll. The contacts on the inner thighs are reflexes for the throat area. The contacts on the outer thighs release the back of the neck and the sides. The shoulder muscles tense and relax during the rocking movement. Stone says:

> The exercise not only releases all the chest muscles involved in breathing and in heart trouble, but also the trapezius muscles which are supplied by the spinal accessory nerves which are the eleventh pair of cranial nerves and the only ones which innervate a muscle. The psoas magnus and the iliacus muscles are also exercised. (Stone, *Polarity Therapy Vol. 2*, p. 47.)

This posture is specifically recommended for rebuilding after heart trouble.

Method

Begin with a reflexology evaluation of the neck. Feel the outer neck and then the throat areas for tender spots. The outer neck area is related to the outer sides of the thigh, and the throat to the inner thighs. The thigh area near the knee is a reflex to the top of the neck near the occiput, while the thigh area near the hip relates to the bottom of the neck near the

Neck-Thigh Relationships

Hold the thighs higher or lower according to whether neck soreness is more high or low.

shoulder. Midway on the thigh relates to midway up the neck.

With this general mapping in mind, see what correspondence you can feel between soreness above and below. Place the hands on the sore spot on the thigh that corresponds to the sore area of the neck and hold these spots firmly. The arms can be crossed or uncrossed, according to which position is more comfortable.

Rocking V

The leg movement is like the pumping action on a playground swing.

To strengthen the abdominal muscles, stop at the V shape instead of coming all the way back up to a sitting position.

Next is a rocking motion. The movement is continuous and smooth and takes some practice. Sit on the floor with knees bent and legs crossed at the ankles. Rock back and pull the legs up, knees coming closer to the chest. Let the head rest on the floor for a moment, neck relaxed, while the legs finish their movement toward the chest. Then extend the legs to rock the body up and forward again, ready to rock back again. Repeat for twenty or more cycles, until you feel a release of tension on the sore spots on the thighs. The legs move in a continuous smooth circular motion throughout the exercise.

Develop these movements into a graceful and smooth self-perpetuating cycle, circling the legs to bring yourself back and up. Continue to firmly grasp the thighs on the sore spots, with arms either uncrossed or crossed, depending on which is easier for your preferred contact location. Feel how the movement releases the tight spots in the thighs. When complete, take a few moments of rest. Then check the areas on the neck to feel the changes.

Variations

The Rocking V may also be done with an emphasis on the hands pulling the thighs up, rather than the legs lifting with abdominal and back muscles. This gives a more stimulating friction-touch to the thighs and activates the brachial plexus muscles.

Benefits
- Tension in the neck and throat area is released, affecting expression.
- The chest is expanded, breathing improved, and the pelvic area is exercised.
- Colon function is stimulated by contact on colon reflex areas on the thighs.
- Tones abdominal muscles; good as a gradual strengthener in ongoing exercise programs.
- Develops heart stability and rhythm.

• Tones the muscles of the back.
• Stimulates energy circulation in the craniosacral pathway.

References

Stone, R. *Polarity Therapy Vol. 2*, pp. 57-58.
Francis, John. *Polarity Self-Help Exercises*, pp. 24-25.
Seidman, Maruti. *A Guide to Polarity Therapy*, p. 139.

Related Exercises

Other exercises influence the neck and shoulders, but have been located elsewhere based on their primary action. To make full use of the book, skip around to note these others and remember them in planning your exercise routine.

Pierre Ha Breath (p. 80)
Woodchopper (p. 84)
Pyramid (p. 97)
Light Rocking Perineal (p. 113)
Rowing (p. 118)
Sympathetic Balance (p. 81)

Chest & Heart

The chest and heart area has a special significance in energy exercises. Stone depicted "the tree of life" with its roots in the chest and branches in the head. The chest is described as:

> ...the sensory root system of feeling through the heart center condensing the finer life currents of sound energy and beating it out in rhythmic pulsations. (Stone, *Polarity Therapy Vol. 2*, p. 19.)

The heart is also the central conductor of the fundamental Yin and Yang energies of the body, and the neutral balancer for the body's positive (head) and negative (pelvis) poles:

> The outward and inward currents must move in all fields if there is to be health and happiness... The heart center is the pivot for the circulation of these energies through the blood... and becomes the control center for these energies. (Stone, *Polarity Therapy Vol. 1 Book 3*, p. 36.)

A gateway to the powers of comprehension above, the heart center is the collector of feelings from below. It is the central conductor of love, expressed in the voice above, the arms to the side, and the pelvis below.

Alexander Lowen offers these comments:

> I have discussed the heart at some length because it is central to all therapy. People come to therapy with various complaints: depression, anxiety, a feeling of inadequacy, a sense of failure, etc. But behind each complaint is a lack of joy and satisfaction in living. It is popular today to talk of self-realization and the human potential, but such terms are meaningless unless one asks, potential for what? If one wants to live more fully and more richly, it is possible only if one opens one's heart to life and to love... The goal

of all therapy is to help a person increase his capacity to give and receive love -- to expand his heart, not just his mind.[10]

The thymus gland near the heart plays an important role. Diamond describes the thymus as a "control room" for the meridians, monitoring the body's flow of Life Force:

> ...the thymus is the first organ of the body to be affected by stress. It is also the first organ to be affected at an energy level by an emotional state. The thymus gland may therefore be thought of as the link between mind and body.[11]

Emotional and psychological difficulties are immediately reflected in the muscles and connective tissue of the chest and heart area. Hardness, rigidity, a concave or slumping posture, over-expansion and other indicators are valuable clues to inner conditions. Emotions relating to desire are centered here, including hope, ambition and greed.

---

[10] Lowen, Alexander. *Bioenergetics*. p. 88-89. While we quote frequently and respectfully from Lowen, there are significant differences between his system and the Polarity model. Lowen's valuable work has roots in the pioneering psychological teachings of Wilhelm Reich. From a Polarity framework, Bioenergetics seems to emphasize the involutionary, Yang half of human experience. "The capacity for pleasure and joy of living," sexual fulfillment, and grounding are frequently-cited goals of therapy; these are all functions of the involutionary side of the "Journey of the Soul." In Polarity, equal concern is accorded the Yin, evolutionary force. Expressions of caution against the common excesses of Yang (irresponsible sex, over-expression of anger, etc.) are more likely to be found in Polarity, and a larger, spiritual context is emphasized. Nevertheless, Lowen eloquently expresses important ideas in the energy field, based on long experience, and he is a valuable resource for the Polarity practitioner.

[11] Diamond, John. *Your Body Doesn't Lie*. p. 62.

11. Taoist Arch

Versions of this pose are found in many sources. We have adopted Lowen's title from *Bioenergetics*. The position is taken naturally when we arise and have a good stretch in the morning, another example of Energy Exercises often being the conscious practice of natural, everyday positions. Young children naturally reach out with both arms as an expression of love. For exercise classes or other group activities, this is a great way to begin, with a joyful reach out to the world.

The posture embodies the attitude of the evolutionary Yin side of the energy cycle. In the first part of the cycle (Yang), the body folds inward as it becomes involved (as embodied in the fetal position or the squat), looking for expression and materialization. Then, as consciousness progresses in the second part of the cycle (Yin), the attention turns back out. The body unfolds in a outward reach as it looks to heaven for greater understanding. Stone describes this turning back to the source as a most important event in the "Journey of the Soul" (see page 237).

Taoist Arch

Method

Stand with your feet shoulder-width apart, or any comfortable pose. Bend the torso back, looking upward, without excessive strain. Reach the arms out fully to the front, the sides and behind the lower back. Breathe fully, exhaling with a deep sigh of satisfaction or a warm expression of greeting and enthusiasm.

Similar benefits can be attained through backward-arch poses such as resting across a fitness ball or a foam roller.

Benefits
- A general toning posture for all dimensions: physical, emotional and mental.
- One of the easiest ways to activate the receptive, evolutionary energy of the Yin Principle.
- Excellent for emotional processing, especially for people with a collapsed chest or slumping shoulders. This can be dramatic and forceful when the pose is held for a minute or more.

References
Lowen, Alexander. *Bioenergetics*, p. 72.
Berkson, Devaki. *The Foot Book*, p. 136.
Diamond, John. *Your Body Doesn't Lie*, p. 57.
Gach, Michael. *Acu-Yoga*, pp. 53, 69, 166.

Related Exercises
Pierre Ha Breath (p. 80)
Cliffhanger (p. 40)
Lion Roar (p. 71)
Thymus Thump (p. 162)
Foot Reflexology (p. 7, 47)

Also see the exercises in these groups:
Shoulders (p. 57)
Diaphragm (p. 87)
Breathing (p. 184)

Diaphragm

The diaphragm is a large dome-shaped muscle in the center of the torso, at the lower edge of the rib cage, separating the thoracic and abdominal body cavities.

While it is relatively unknown to many beginners, the diaphragm has great importance in energy movement. With the brachial plexus (the nerve group which starts in the neck and extends down to the shoulder blades), it supplies part of the force necessary for breathing, while also supporting the heart from below.

Stone considered the diaphragm to be especially important because it represents the neutral, transitional link between Yang (above) and Yin (below). On a physical level, hardness and rigidity of the diaphragm is associated with shallow breathing and reduced vitality.

> The diaphragm is the main respiratory muscle doing the most important work in life. Every cell needs the life energy contained in the breath... Truly the diaphragm is the firmament which divides the energy above and below... It is the bridge where mind and life cross into the emotional vital field. (Stone, *Polarity Therapy Vol. 1*, Book 2, p. 35.)

> The diaphragm is the elastic, functioning firmament which divides the waters or energies, above from below. It divides the two rivers above (one the Fire and the other the Air Element) from the two rivers (the Earth Element and the Water Element) below. It is upon this important interaction that life depends. Without diaphragmatic function, there can be no respiration nor heart beat, no proper assimilation nor elimination, nor motion. It is a fixed stabilizer of bodily function. (Stone, *Polarity Therapy Vol. 1*, Book 1, p. 25.)

From its central position in the torso, the diaphragm supports and massages the internal organs, moves the lymph and aids digestion.

On an emotional level, diaphragm therapies have been valuable for those experiencing an inability to give and take freely, communicate deeply and sincerely, take bold action or fully engage in relationships.

> When the diaphragm is free, the heart is free to act without fear or apprehension. (Stone, *Polarity Therapy Vol. 2*, p. 46.)

When a person is under emotional stress, tightness of the diaphragm indicates a tendency to implode or explode rather than being able to communicate successfully.

The diaphragm is also considered a gateway to the solar plexus, center of power in the body. Thus diaphragm exercises are ideal for developing the ability to manifest power in a balanced way, neither tyrant nor wimp archetype. It is associated with the Fire Element and its functions of action, authority, digestion and force.

Other authors' comments on the diaphragm:

"...the diaphragm is the gateway through which feelings generated in the lower three chakras pass as they move to the upper portions of the bodymind."

– Ken Dychtwald, *Bodymind*, p. 141.

"Diaphragm: This muscle comes up approximately 95% of the time as the priority muscle in body/mind integration."

– Frank Mahoney, *Hyperton-x*, p. 38.

"It is the thorax [which is centered on the diaphragm] which connects the source of power, our pelvis, with our head, the source of orientation and intentional movement. The link doesn't work, and the reason is that we never did actually try to do what we wanted. We always did what somebody found right for us... Ida Rolf understood this. For she made her first lesson, not on the head, nor on the pelvis, but here at the link, and if you ask why... [it is because] she felt she had been trying to find the most effective way to start."

– Moshe Feldenkrais, *The Master Moves*, p. 78.

---

12. Diaphragm Reflexes

The web of the hand, the top edge of the foot's long arch (just below the ball of the foot), and the front part of the forearm just above the elbow are commonly used reflexes for the diaphragm. Additionally, all joints (ankle, knee, hip, wrist, elbow and shoulder) are diaphragm reflexes often used in Polarity Therapy, and are incorporated in many exercises. As we did with the shoulders, it is useful to first press on the diaphragm with the fingertips, to get a feeling for its tension, then do some reflexology, then repeat the test. Typically, the diaphragm muscle will be dramatically relaxed after a reflexology treatment.

A secondary area for the diaphragm is along the lines which form between the corners of the mouth and outsides of

Diaphragm Reflexes

The thumb web and elbow joint are good diaphragm release reflexes. Having a helper hold both points at once, below right, is extra-effective.

the nose, below the cheek bones. Nearby reflex points slightly higher, in the cheeks below the eyes, are linked to the thymus gland. These areas are naturally stimulated by smiling and laughing, perhaps a factor in the benefits of laughter in therapy, such as ideas popularized by Norman Cousins.

Method

Use your fingers to find tense or sore spots in any of the reflex areas described above. Press in lightly or deeply, depending on your personal preference and the circumstances: a light touch will be soothing and balancing, while a deeper pressure will create change. Push in and hold for a count of at least 8, waiting for a softening of tissues signaling release. You can also use a circular moving pressure with the fingertips or thumb for a more stimulating effect.

After pressure on a reflex, experiment with a balancing contact. Place one hand on the reflex and the other on the diaphragm area and hold lightly. Often the energy balancing effect can be perceived as a pulse in the fingertips or a wave-like sensation of relaxation.

Benefits

- Releases the diaphragm without direct contact. In bodywork, reflex techniques are often used to prepare the target area for direct contact.
- Useful for digestive pains, gas and hiccoughs. For hiccoughs, the web of the hand is particularly useful; use deep pressure without undue pain and allow several minutes.
- Useful to facilitate communication and overcome anxiety.
- Facilitates processing of emotions relating to anger and authority.

References

Stone, R. *Polarity Therapy Vol. 1*, Book 2, p. 11.
Stone, R. *Polarity Therapy Vol. 2*, pp. 35-42,183-184.
Diamond, John. *Your Body Doesn't Lie*, pp. 89-94.

13. Calf Reflex

A multiple reflex is found in the calves. The calves are the neutral zone in the lower part of the body just as the diaphragm area is the neutral zone in the middle part (see chart on page 27). The calves also have specific reflex relationships with the chest (linked by the Neutral Principle) and the colon (linked by the Earth Element). Stone discusses contacts on the calves in relation to elimination of waste gas from the body and improved digestive function. The same concept appears in the Dennisons' "Foot Flex" contact found on page 115.

Method

Take a kneeling position, resting the buttocks back on the calves. Make the hand into a fist, lift up for a moment, and place the fist on the calf muscle. Now lower the buttocks down, creating pressure on the calf from the knuckles of the fist. Make a strong "a-a-a-h-h-h" sound as you exhale. Hold for a moment, then lift and move the hands to a new spot. The sorest spots offer the most benefit.

In addition to the calves, this same kneeling position is a good stance for reflex treatment of the feet. Continue down from the calves, pressing the Achilles tendon, then the ankle, then down the bottom of the foot. This is a good general treatment, and very enjoyable in a class setting, with lots of good-natured moaning and groaning.

References

Seigel, Alan. *Polarity Therapy*, pp. 100-101.
Francis, John. *Polarity Self-Help Exercises*, p. 39.

14. Diaphragm Press

This exercise combines conscious breathing with direct pressure of the fingers on the diaphragm. It is effective for opening the diaphragm, and also affects the pelvic area. The diaphragm and pelvis are linked physiologically by the psoas muscle (the muscle we use to lift the legs when we walk), which attaches to the spine at the diaphragm level.

This posture is an easier variation of the Diaphragm Press-Leg Lift, which is described next. It was devised to give diaphragm contact without strenuous leg lifting, which is to be avoided by some people with back weaknesses.

Method

Kneel on a soft surface or sit in a chair. Place the backs of the fingers of both hands together, fingers straight, to make a "wedge." With the fingers, push up and in lightly about one and a half inches below the ribs. In the very middle of the rib cage and below the sternum is the xiphoid process, a cartilage structure: make sure that you are well below or to the side of this projection, as it should not be stressed. Check for tense areas. Once you have a sense of the current state of tension, begin the release process.

Pick a tight spot and place your fingertips there. Inhale, and as you exhale, lean forward to allow the fingers to sink in. Keep the fingers at that level of penetration and inhale into them to create more pressure. As you exhale, lean forward again, and allow the fingers to sink in further. This process can continue for some time, gradually going deeper with each breath.

Diaphragm Press

This kneeling position is also used for calf reflex work (make fists and sandwich them between calf and thigh as you sit back) and also for the self-organ drain (page 70). The same hand position is used in other diaphragm press positions including standing and prone.
This may be stressful if the knees are weak or injured. All these exercises can be done sitting or standing, if needed for knee comfort.

Benefits
- The diaphragm relaxes, facilitating a wider range of expansion and contraction.
- Breathing, digestion, and heart functions are supported and enhanced.
- The torso, from shoulders above to pelvis below, is lengthened and relaxed.
- Beneficial as a part of bodywork therapies dealing with dissociation of mind and body, or self and feelings.
- Enhances communication.
- Primary energy circuits passing through the diaphragm area are opened.
- Assists in the movement of gas.
- Eases problems of fear or low confidence.
- Balances left/right, front/back and top/bottom energy dimensions.

Reference

Stone, R. *Polarity Therapy Vol. 2*, pp. 47-49.

15. Diaphragm Activation

The activation technique is useful for the diaphragm, accessing the deeper connections of the diaphragm to the spine and ribs. This activation helps the breath and diaphragm to reset at a wider range of motion, restoring ease to the breathing cycle.

Method

Place both hands flat on the stomach area, with the thumbs just high enough to touch the lowest ribs. Inhale and exhale a few times to experience and become familiar with your breathing pattern. Then inhale fully and hold your breath. As you hold, push gently against the upper belly with your fingertips, and push your belly against your hands. The muscle is internal, so the activation of it is largely through holding the breath. When you feel that you need to, press the belly out as you exhale. Pause and experience how your breathing cycle feels now. This can be repeated several times.

Benefits
• Provides relief when breathing has become shallow and restricted.

References

Mahoney, Frank. *Hyperton-x*, p. 40.

Dennison, Paul and Gail. *Brain Gym*, p. 10.

Barhydt, Harrison and Elizabeth. *Self-Help for Stress and Pain*, p. 43.

16. Diaphragm Press Leg Lift

This is a continuation of the diaphragm press described earlier. The purpose of lifting the legs is to stimulate the diaphragm by flexing the psoas muscle, which attaches to the spine at the diaphragm level.

The original exercise described by Stone is now rarely used: leg lifts have been found to be stressful for the back. The original is described under "Variations" for those whose back fitness is excellent. Instructors are advised to be very

Diaphragm Press Leg Lift and Variations   *Lower back*

The upper picture shows the main posture; the lower picture shows a variation that is easier to do and also safer for sore backs.

Caution

sensitive to the fitness level of all students in the class before using the old-fashioned straight leg lift posture.

Method

Lie on the back and again use the fingertips to check under the ribs for tension. As before, be careful not to press directly on the xiphoid process. Place the fingertips on the spot of your choice, or wherever feels most tense along the diaphragm.

Leg lifting movements are combined with a specific sequence of breathing. First, inhale fully with the legs resting. Then, as you exhale, lift one straight leg and allow the fingers to press into the diaphragm area. Inhale again, maintaining that fingertip pressure on the diaphragm. As you exhale, bend the leg, allowing the knee to come toward the chest while the fingers sink in. Inhale, maintaining that same level of penetration with the fingertips into the diaphragm, and breathe into the fingers. Exhale again and allow the fingers to sink in further. Relax in this position, and repeat the inhale/rest-without-backing-off, and exhale/press-in-deeper sequences until you are ready to stop.

When you feel ready to complete this leg lift, inhale while straightening the leg; exhale while lowering the leg and allowing the fingers to sink in. Relax and keep your hands at that level of pressure for a while.

To finish, take the fingertips out and let them rest gently on the diaphragm area for a short time, at least one third of the time that was spent doing the posture.

After resting, repeat the sequence for the other leg.

Variations

This leg lift may also be done from a starting position of feet resting on the floor and both knees bent. Inhale. Exhale and lift both bent legs at once, allowing the fingers to sink into the diaphragm area. Continue as above.

A person with strong abdominal muscles and a strong back can lift both straight legs at once as shown on page 68. This is the way the exercise was originally presented by Stone. However, this may be unsafe for the average person.

In addition, a standing position variation is offered by John Francis. In this posture, the fingertips are placed in the diaphragm area and the torso is lowered, head to the knees, with a slow "ahhh" sound. In the collapsed position, the fingertips can press in more deeply.

Benefits
• Same as Diaphragm Press.

References
Stone, R. *Polarity Therapy Vol. 2*, pp. 55-56
Francis, *Polarity Self-Help Exercises*, pp. 40-41.

17. Organ Drain
This is an easy way to activate and "massage" the organs of the abdominal cavity, especially the intestines and colon. It is grouped with diaphragm exercises because they have a common effect in digestive function, and because it can be used for relaxation after a strenuous diaphragm press exercise. It also helps deal with difficulties in the lower back (often lower back problems originate with emotional or digestive tension in front) or pelvis (problems in areas that support the abdominal area create problems in the area itself).

Method
In a kneeling position, leaning over the knees (as shown in the illustration for the Diaphragm Press on p. 66), use the fingertips to gently explore the abdominal area. Press in with small circular motions. Start on the lower right corner above the hip, and gradually work up and across, then down the left side, repeating as desired. If a particular spot is painful, reduce the pressure.

This can also be done by holding in one place in the ab-domen, exhaling, and then inhaling into the spot being held. Gentle rotational pressure can then be used.

This exercise is based on Stone's "Gas Releasing Tech-nique."

Benefits
• Gives relief from gas pains.
• Tones the internal connective tissues.
• Can be helpful with sluggish bowels.

References
Stone, R. *Polarity Therapy Vol. 1*, Book 3, pp. 93-94.
Stone, R. *Health Building*, p. 178.

18. Lion Roar

The Lion Roar uses sound to expand and project the heat of the solar plexus. The roaring sound is a deep, full, continuous emptying of the lungs, vibrating the body from the inside out and opening the diaphragm. The rich, loud sound is quite exhilarating, giving the same therapeutic warmth we feel when singing in a choral group or yelling at a sports event. The Lion Roar is a specific therapy for those wishing to strengthen or activate the ability to express feelings, safely expel pent-up frustration, or strengthen Yang qualities such as creativi-ty, responsibility and assertiveness.

Method
Take a position in which you can comfortably place your elbows between your knees with hands clasped in the middle. Make sure your chest is open. There are several possibilities for this po-sition, the best being the Squat (page 101).

Lion Roar

Lion Roar Variations

First, take one or more cleansing breaths. Inhale deeply through the nose and exhale fully. Now you are ready for the "roar." Inhale, expanding the chest, and as you exhale, let the breath out with a roaring sound that is full and rich.

Make a deep, low, relaxed sound for maximum volume with minimal strain. If there is strain, reduce the loudness. Once there is an easy, steady tone, increase the volume again. Be aware of and avoid the tendency to pinch or constrict the throat. While you roar, push the hands together and the knees into the elbows (a double diaphragm reflex connection), and focus the eyes (the positive pole of the Yang Principle) on a specific spot. Expel the breath to the last drop. This may be followed with more deep breaths and roars (three roars is a good total for most people) until you feel that frustrations are exhausted and warmth is shining through.

After the roars, move into a balancing posture by placing both thumbs between the eyebrows. This is Stone's "Youth Posture," depicted on p. 138 of *Health Building*. Take a few moments to feel the inner energy level, the heat of the solar plexus, tingling in the hands and face, increased ability to express feelings and deeper breathing ability.

Variations

When you are in a situation in which it is not appropriate to be noisy, this posture may be done with a muted long deep forceful exhalation.

Also in this posture, a general toning exercise for the face may be added by "making faces" in all directions, activating the facial muscles. Stick out the tongue as far as possible, open the jaw as wide as possible, raise and lower the eyebrows, purse the lips, etc. The face is a complex field of reflexes for the whole body and this expression-making is both relaxing and fun.

Benefits
- Multiple reflex connections facilitate general energy balancing.
- Hands clasped and squeezing relates to shoulders and brachial plexus.
- Elbows touching knees makes a diaphragm reflex connection.
- Belly touching thighs connects neutral and negative poles of the Fire Element and stimulates the body's heat or fire.
- Releases pent-up frustrations and aids digestion. This can be very useful in emotional processing during therapy.
- Improves the free flow of expression.

References
The Lion Roar originates in Hatha Yoga; this version is described by Stone in discussing the Squat (*Health Building*, p. 138, 163).
Francis, John. *Polarity Self-Help Exercises*, p. 22.
Berkson, Devaki. *The Foot Book*, pp. 180-181.

19. Ha Breath

Stone used a sound called the "Ha Breath" in several exercises. To introduce these, we first introduce the sound itself. The "Ha" sound takes a little practice for beginners. The sound is full and forceful and comes from deep in the belly, vibrating the whole torso as it comes out.

Begin to develop this sound by placing your hands on the belly just below the diaphragm. If you are making the sound properly, you will feel your hands move as the "ha" comes out. A "ho ho ho" like Santa Claus is a fun way to get started. As you feel the belly move, give the sound some extra length following a forceful "h-h-h-a-a-a." Play with this. It will feel easy and natural and make a full deep sound as you do it correctly and the diaphragm opens. When done properly, the sound is loud, bouncing out effortlessly and filling the room. It combines power with ease, and should not require straining. Instructors can take time to help the class feel comfortable with making a rich "h-h-h-a-a-a" sound.

20. Up and Down Ha Breath

This is the first and best known of the Ha Breath postures. Stone called this the "Exercise for Polarizing the Energy Currents," an indication of its multiple values for all parts of the energy anatomy.

The primary effect of the Ha Breath is on the Fire Element center, located in the solar plexus. It can be described as the stoking and heating of a furnace, in which the solar plexus represents the fireplace containing hot embers, the brachial plexus and chest represents the air supply, and the thighs represent the fuel. All parts of the system are activated and stimulated by the movements, generating increased circulation and power.

In addition to its effect on the Fire systems, this Ha Breath is also stimulating to the pelvic area (the Yin Principle and Water Element), and the diaphragm (the Neutral Principle). To continue the furnace analogy, the pelvis is like a water basin. Heated by the increased action of the nearby thighs, the pelvic basin's contents of old feelings are activated and moved upward across the diaphragm towards expression at the throat. Self-expression is a significant form of release or elimination; the Ha Breath stimulates the expressive pathway.

In addition, the upper back is activated by the position and action of the arms and hands. Thus the Ha Breath is one of the most stimulating and comprehensive of all Stone's exercises.

This movement is one of several of Stone's postures that have proven to be useful in bodywork. The more stimulating exercises accomplish energy activation that can be difficult for a therapist to induce without deep contact. The Ha Breath, Pyramid, Cliffhanger, Woodchopper and others can be used to quickly increase energy circulation without using deep contact.

Like the Cliffhanger, the Up and Down Ha Breath needs to be be done with caution. For those with sore knees or backs, it can be modified to reduce the movement.

Method

To do the Ha Breath, stand with the legs slightly more than shoulder-width apart. Lean forward so the hands rest on the knees, fingers conveniently aligning vertically with the energy pathways of the Long Lines Current or Yin Principle.

From this partially-bent position, slowly lower the body to the position shown in the illustration, letting out a deep full "Ha" sound as you go. Relax your neck (everyone will need to be repeatedly reminded of this), and bend with the legs, not the waist. The back stays straight, almost parallel to

Ha Breath: Up and Down Positions

Caution
✳
Lower back, Knees

the floor, and the head stays down in the lowered position. The chest opens and closes as the arms push up and down: this activates the chest and diaphragm, creating a bellows effect to fan the flames of the solar plexus.

From the lowered position, push (hands on thighs just above the knees) back up to the upright position as shown in the illustration. The arms, not the legs, should be doing the lifting work: you should be able to feel movement in the shoulder blades. Once up, drop down again with another strong "Ha" sound. Remember to relax your neck. Repeat this as many times as feels appropriate for your body and the situation. If you are seeking relief from angry feelings or wanting to dramatically increase or discharge your fiery qualities, the Up and Down Ha Breath can be done repeatedly.

Variations

For an easier variation, sit in a chair with the legs more than shoulder width apart, hands on knees as described above. Proceed the same as above, but adjust your movements to suit the limits of sitting in the chair. Remember to push with the arms as you come up and make a nice full "Ha" as you go down. As always, remember to relax your neck. This is a way for seniors and those with weak knees or back to benefit from the exercise.

An advanced variation uses the same up and down movements but with the arms behind the back, hands clasped as shown in the illustration on page 107. This creates a dramatic opening across the front of the chest area.

Benefits
- Stimulating for physical and emotional energy levels. One of the most comprehensive self-given "Energy Session" exercises, with both top-bottom (Yin Principle) and front-back (Yang Principle) balancing effects.
- Relief from gas.
- Relief from nervousness.
- Opens diaphragm.

- Tones back, especially lower back.
- Relaxes muscles around the brachial plexus.
- Fire is activated by sound and by thigh action.
- Brings what is inside to the surface.
- Expansive sound frees expression.

References
Stone, R. *Health Building*, p. 162.
Stone, R. *Polarity Therapy Vol. 2*, p. 191.
Sills, Franklyn. *The Polarity Process*, p. 153.
Seidman, Maruti. *A Guide to Polarity Therapy*, p. 137.
Francis, John. *Polarity Self-Help Exercises*, p. 19.

21. Sciatic Ha Breath

Sciatic Ha Breath is a demanding but beneficial releasing exercise for the lower back and legs, especially the hamstrings and Sciatic nerve. It retains the up and down movement of the regular Ha Breath, but is much slower, with a groaning slow sound instead of the forceful Ha. For acute sciatica, the Sciatic Ha Breath can be too strenuous.

Method
Stand with feet about ten inches apart, toes turning inward. Bend over and grasp the heels with the hands, pulling down to lengthen the lower back. For most people, this re-

**Sciatic
Ha Breath**

Caution
✳
Lower back

quires bending the knees; flexible people will need to straighten the knees and bend the elbows, keeping chest to thigh as the legs straighten. Inhale as you bend the knees, making it easier to hold the ankle, then straighten the legs as you exhale with a steady groaning sound. The effect is an activation for the back of the legs, isometrically opposed by the arms gripping the heels.

Benefits

- Lengthens muscles around the sciatic nerve and back of the legs.
- Improves posture, especially problems with tilted pelvis and stressed sacrum area.
- Integrates and balances the top and bottom of the body, the path of the Yin Principle.
- Useful for developing flexibility with Yang challenges such as using authority and making decisions.
- Lengthens the back. Grasping the back of the ankle stimulates the Achilles heel reflex to the lower back. The fingertips press the inside of the ankle, a reflex to the pelvis and emotional history (see hallucis tendon, page 95).

22. Arch Pull Ha Breath

The Arch Pull Ha Breath is another advanced variation, which specifically lengthens and tones the lower back and thighs. Like the Sciatic Ha, it is strenuous. The movement is an isometric pull with a slow groaning sound. It should be approached cautiously by those with knee or back pain.

The Arch Pull Ha Breath resembles both the regular Ha Breath and the Squat (page 101). Its unique feature is the placement of the hands under the arches, a reflex connection for the umbilicus and solar plexus.

This neutral position of the body is completed with the hands under the arches of the feet, so the Polarity Currents can be completed and flow freely.

Method

Bend over and place the hands under the arches of the feet. Breathe in, then pull with the hands to lower the body down to a Squat position with a groaning "Ha" exhalation. The hands pull on the arches throughout the movement. While pulling down, resist with the legs; while moving down, resist with the arms. The greater the resistance, the greater the heat generated. After a few up-and-down movements, stay down in the squat position and rock gently from front to back, then side to side, then in circles. Continue breathing fully, with a groaning "Ha" sound on each exhalation. Again, remember to keep pulling on the arches throughout the exercise.

Arch Pull Ha Breath

Caution
*
Lower back

Benefits

- Beneficial for Yang Principle systems, including back muscles, solar plexus, and thighs, which are the negative pole of the Fire Element; generates intense heat.
- Stimulates the front-back dimension of the torso. This dimension is also the path of the Umbilical Current or Yang Principle.
- Counters nervousness.
- Good for releasing gas.
- Strengthens pelvic muscles.
- Tones thighs and back.

References

Stone, R. *Polarity Therapy Vol. 2*, p. 193.
Stone, R. *Health Building*, pp. 162-163, 171.

23. Pierre Ha Breath

This dynamic Ha Breath was devised by Pierre Pannetier, ND (1910-1984), Stone's student and protégé. Most people are able to do it easily, and it is fun for groups or classes. It makes use of a technique called "Crossing Over" which appears in several other Polarity Therapy movements. Passing the arms or legs back and forth across each other stimulates energy flow and balance. An analogy for this is the dynamo, which generates electricity by revolving a magnet within a magnetic field, "crossing over" the magnetic poles.

In terms of energy theory, this movement accentuates the Neutral Principle, the side-to-side movement of energy throughout the body. This dimension of energy is activated simultaneously by several movements here: the opening and stretching of the "air oval" in the chest for greater breathing, the opening of the diaphragm muscle through the "Ha" sound, and the activation of chest and diaphragm reflexes while lifting up on the balls of the feet for the "Ha." The active movement, strong sound and rhythmic repetition combine to make a stimulating, light hearted exercise.

The Pierre Ha exercise is a dynamic version of the evolutionary Taoist Arch pose, described earlier (p. 59). Moving the arms forcefully back and projecting the chest opens the heart area and stimulates the thymus. Thus this exercise could be grouped with the chest area exercises, with the functions and benefits described there.

Method

Begin with some warm-up movements for the shoulders and neck. Stand with the feet a comfortable, supportive distance apart. Practice lifting up to the balls of the feet to check your balance and stability. Make a practice "Ha" sound or two and then add a crossover arm movement. Put the arms out in front with the palms facing up. Cross them quickly by moving right over left, left over right, right over left three

Pierre
Ha Breath

times (see illustrations) and then swing them back briskly with a loud "Ha!" The timing of the Ha! is important; it should be at the point of fullest extension. If it is just right, the sound will pop out effortlessly. The exercise takes on a "1-2-3-Ha!" rhythm. Now add rising up on the balls of the feet (a reflex for the chest) as you reach the "ha" in the movement. This can take a little practice, but it is fun and easy to do. Remember to take a quiet moment standing after completion, eyes closed, knees slightly bent, to experience the results of the exercise.

Variations

For those with stiff shoulders, it is not necessary to have the palms facing upwards, and preliminary warm-ups may be necessary. The arm activation techniques described earlier can be good for this.

For the Pierre Ha Breath, here's a quick activation warm-up. With the arms straight out to the sides and thumbs pointing up, inhale and "float" the arms backward. Exhale and push against an imaginary force that holds the arms from going forward. Inhale and let the arms float back again. Repeat this as long as the arms' range of motion keeps increasing, then allow them to float forward and rest. This isometric technique may also be done pressing against a doorway or wall, and is especially helpful for people whose shoulders curve forward excessively.

Benefits
- Energizing, relaxing and fun for a group.
- Opens the chest, shoulders, breathing, diaphragm.
- Brings alertness and clarity of thought.
- Good for postural slumping shoulder problems.
- Balances the side-to-side Neutral Principle.

24. Side To Side Ha Breath

The Side To Side Ha Breath is highly popular for many reasons. It is very effective, giving a direct experience of energy flow to many who try it. It is also easy to do and is thus well-suited to classes for seniors and/or beginners.

In energy theory, this version adds a stimulation to the Transverse Current (side-to-side, Neutral Principle) to go with the Long-line current (Bi-Polar, Yin Principle) effect of the Up and Down Ha Breath. As always, the "Ha" sound stimulates the front/back dimension of the Yang Principle.

Caution

✳

Lower back

**Side to Side
Ha Breath**

Method

Begin in a standing position, feet 24 inches or so apart. Lean forward to place the hands on the knees, keeping the back straight. So far this posture is similar to the Pyramid, and the two can be mistaken in Stone's illustrations. Here, however, the weight of the torso is never transferred fully to the arms/shoulders. Instead, the weight is evenly distributed between arms and legs.

From this position, begin the Ha Breath sequence by moving smoothly to place the chest down on one thigh as you exhale with a "H-a-a-a" sound. From the low position, chest on one thigh, inhale and use the arms to raise the torso back to center, then exhale and go down to the other side, chest on thigh again with a "H-a-a-a" sound. The upper body makes an arc, from one knee to the other.

We have experimented with a wide range of sounds and tempos here, soft and slow for relaxation, loud and forceful for stimulation; experiment to determine the sound and speed that is right for you. Repeat several cycles to feel the benefits.

Benefits
- Good posture for feeling energy movement.
- General energy balancing for all major systems; especially appropriate for left-right Neutral Principle imbalances.
- Can be soothing or stimulating, according to tempo and volume of movement and sound and the amount of pressure exerted by the hands on the legs.
- Gentle spinal stretch, suitable for all ages (can be done in a chair).
- Soothing internal massage for the abdominal cavity.
- Facilitates movement and elimination of gas.

References
Stone, R. *Health Building*, pp. 160-161.
Francis, John. *Polarity Self-Help Exercises*, p. 20.

25. Woodchopper

The Woodchopper could be located in many sections of this book, since it affects the whole system. It emphasizes connecting top and bottom, and stimulating the back side and Fire Element energies. It is an advanced and strenuous technique and should be avoided by those with back problems.

The Woodchopper is a forceful, dynamic and fun involutionary-to-evolutionary movement, adding action to the positions of the Taoist Arch and the Squat. It also resembles the Rocking Cliff (page 38) in embodying the involution/evolution positions.

Method

For safety, warm up for the Woodchopper by lengthening and movement. Key areas are the hamstrings, back and pelvis. Stand with feet a little wider than the shoulders, knees

Woodchopper

Caution
✱
Lower back

slightly bent. From a standing position, hang down and let the arms swing freely like an elephant's trunk. Then stand with hands on hips and rotate the pelvis, like a hula dancer. Place the hands on the hips and practice the up-and-down movement: pelvis forward, then back, as the chest expands forward then falls to the knees in a smooth motion. The hands-on-hip variation is safer because there is less leverage on the back. Other warm-ups for the Woodchopper are Rowing (p. 118), Hamstring Lengthening (p. 202) and the Pierre Ha Breath (p. 80).

The movement is a natural swinging motion as if holding an axe and chopping wood. Starting with hands clasped and reaching high above the head, rock the pelvis forward to start an undulating swing which goes all the way down and through the legs. Let out a solid "Ha!" at the end of the stroke. The sound should pop out almost on its own as you reach the bottom. This movement can be repeated many times, taking on a rhythmic feeling. The effect is like a wave which ripples up and down the spine as you swing and return, from pelvis through shoulders and arms. Remember that the movement is generated by the pelvis, not the arms. Be careful to not go too fast, and be moderate in using the Woodchopper. Too much force and speed could lead to dizziness and strain.

Benefits
- Integrates the top-bottom dimension of the Yin Principle.
- Opens the diaphragm, the bridge between upper and lower areas.
- Activates Yang Principle and Fire Element: good for stimulating authority and assertiveness.
- Alternates involutionary Yang (curved in the front) and evolutionary Yin (arched to the back) poses for balancing.
- Grounding: generates a feeling of practicality and a "can-do" attitude.

References
Stone, R. *Health Building*, p. 159.
Stone, R. *Polarity Therapy Vol. 2*, p. 191.
Berkson, Devaki, *The Foot Book*, p. 130.
Francis, John. *Polarity Self-Help Exercises*, pp. 37-38

Lower Back

The lower back is a common region of difficulty for many people. Pains in this area can be frequently traced to tension in the front.

> Abdominal tension and stress are frequently at the root of lower back pain, for as the muscles in the belly tighten and contract, they begin to tug on the muscles which surround the spine, forcing them to become contracted and rigid.[12]

This link between front and back can be described in terms of emotional experience. The Yin front with its stored emotions is a powerful motivator for the action-oriented Yang back. Sensory (front) precedes Motor (back): "The senses open the way and the motor impulses obey." (Stone, *Polarity Therapy Vol. 1*, p. 70.) Our sensory processes guide our motor processes about what to do. Actions undertaken for emotional reasons (compulsive behavior, obsessions, addictions, etc.) are often stressful and exhausting.

In energy anatomy, the lower back is associated with Yang involution, generating new life through sexuality, and involvement through creative action, materialism and power. The sacrum at the base of the spine serves several functions in energy anatomy, including being the center of this involutionary force, the negative pole of the spinal system and the animalistic complement to the higher powers of the brain above. Advanced structural balance techniques in Polarity Therapy analyze the alignment of the sacrum in the pelvic basin to indicate the condition of the body's energy currents.

Obviously the lower back also has major structural significance. Stone described how posture, the presence of a short leg, abnormal gait, spinal curvature and even sinus problems are often related to sacrum/lower back conditions.

---

[12] Dychtwald, Ken. *Bodymind.* p. 27.

26. Back Reflexes

The most commonly used reflexes for the lower part of the torso are found in the heel, achilles tendon and instep. Use light or deep pressure with the fingertips to stimulate and massage these areas. The Achilles tendon is often tight and sore when lower back tension is high. The back of the heel relates specifically to the sacrum.

Along the inside edge of the foot, the spine reflexes range from lower back at the heel to upper back near the toe. The curve of the spine and the inside edge of the foot are similar in shape, making it easy to locate specific corresponding areas.

Back-Foot Relationships
Press along the inside of the foot for spinal reflexes.

Another relaxing reflex area for the back is the ear. Take each hand and pull lightly along the edge of the ear, especially at the bottom, a reflex to the pelvic area. Lift up firmly on the ridge directly above the ear canal. Similarly, the nose is a reflex to the spine and can be lightly pulled downward or moved in a small motion for a relaxing effect: reflexes are arranged from top to bottom corresponding to the area from shoulder to sacrum.

References
- Stone, R. *Polarity Therapy Vol. 1*, Book 2, pp. 11, 24, 38, 40, 79; Book 3, pp. 45-49.
- Stone, R. *Polarity Therapy Vol. 2*, pp. 105-109, 118, 163, 198, 201.
- Berkson, Devaki. *The Foot Book*. p. 56.
- Stokes & Whiteside. *One Brain*, Chapter 8, p. 9.

27. Gluteal Activation

Most people, especially those with tightness in the lower back, have tension in the gluteal muscles. This posture creates a gentle pressure in a direction opposite to that which we actually want to release, to facilitate the lengthening of the gluteal muscles.

Method

Lie on the floor with the legs straight. Slowly slide one heel toward the chest so that the knee comes up to a bent position. Slowly raise that one knee and bring it close to the chest, embracing it with the arms to support its resting position. Take a deep breath in and, as you exhale, push the knee (with about 25% of full force) into the arms. The arms exactly meet the force of the push so there is no resulting movement.

As you inhale, relax your leg and allow the knee to drop more closely to the chest. Do not pull or force, "allow." Take up any slack with your arms and repeat the exhale-push- inhale-relax two more times.

Rest the leg in this new position and allow the body to experience and register this new leg position. This may also be done with the arms between the knee and the calf to affect a slightly different area.

Repeat with the other leg, and then with both legs together. This is a great warm up for the "Back Curl," immediately following, which is done in this position. Another activation which replicates more of the traditional squat is to grasp the feet and activate by pushing with the legs and re-

Gluteal Activation

89

sisting with the hands, similar to the position in Rowing (p. 118), and in the Arch Pull Ha Breath (p. 78).

Benefits
- Relaxes the lower back area.
- Lengthens the gluteal muscles.

Reference
Stone, R. *Health Building*, p. 134.

28. Back Curl

This is a relaxing variation of the Squat that is specific for the back. It is well known in many therapies for relief of back pain. It can be very relaxing in bed as first aid for insomnia and for "unwinding" from a busy day, before sleep. It re-creates the shape of the Squat, without strain on the knees or ankles.

Method

Lie on the floor or bed with the legs out straight. Slowly slide the heels so that the knees come into a bent position (feet still resting on the floor). Slowly raise the knees and bring them close to the chest. Embrace them with the arms. Rock gently from side to side and then stop and relax, feeling the benefits of the posture. As a variation, move the knees from side to side with minimal movement in the back, giving a gentle wringing motion to the back muscles. For a different variation, activation for the back can be done by pressing the legs against the resistance of the arms or hands.

Back Curl

References
Stone, R. *Health Building*, pp. 132-137.
Berkson, Devaki. *The Foot Book*, pp. 87-88.
Lowen, Alexander. *The Way to Vibrant Health*, p. 102.

29. The Clock

This mindful differentiation sequence comes from Moshe Feldenkrais. It works with the spine, spinal muscles, pelvic muscles, neck and the deeper postural muscles in front and back.

Method

Lie on the back with the knees up, feet comfortably apart, hands resting at the sides. Imagine that you are resting on the face of a clock. Gently rock your pelvis toward your feet (toward "6 o'clock") so that the tail bone comes closer to the floor. Now gently and slowly rock your pelvis up the other way (toward "12 o'clock") so that your lower back curve (lumbar spine) moves closer to the floor. The movements are slow and gentle. Only subtle muscle movement is required. Do this "6" to "12" and back to "6" slow rocking motion several times, noticing the movement of the head and chin as well as the pelvis.

Next, begin a slow movement toward "9 o'clock." The knees will move slightly and the weight will shift to the right hip. Return with a movement toward "3 o'clock" and the weight shifts onto the left hip. Do this several times, rest, and begin again. When you have completed these up-down and side-to-side motions, "rock around the clock" very slowly.

Start at "12 o'clock" and do a clockwise rotation, "12-1-2-3-4,"

The Clock

and so on. Observe the difference between the right and left sides. After several times, repeat in the other direction. Let the head move too. Whenever movement doesn't feel smooth and circular, stop and imagine a circular movement.

As a variation, move back and forth between opposite points on the clock: from "12 to 6" and back, then "1 to 7," and so on. Feel how you move and stay comfortable.

References
Feldenkrais, Moshe. *Awareness Through Movement*, p. 115.
Bach-y-Rita, Eileen. "Feldenkrais at Home: Aligning Your Body" (audio).

Pelvis

The pelvic basin is a factor in all structural conditions and energetic pathways. It is significant in all aspects of energy therapy, being the "south pole" of the magnetic field of the torso. Pelvis relaxation is an essential focus of Polarity Therapy; Stone found that pelvic therapies made chiropractic adjustments last longer, and gave insight into the emotional origins of tension.

The pelvis is the foundation of structure, the seat of regeneration, the source of courageous confidence, and the storage vault for old unprocessed feelings. Repeating one of the most frequently-quoted lines from Stone,

> In the pelvic basin at the bottom is the sum total force accumulation of all the sensory tension and emotional frustration. (Stone, *Polarity Therapy Vol. 1, Book 2*, p. 16.)

Therapeutic exercises for the pelvic area can be expected to have a significant impact elsewhere.

> Our experience indicates that the hips are the basic structural element in the body and that balancing the lower back also corrects problems in other areas.[13]

This significance is particularly useful in emotional processing: it is common for old memories and unexpressed feelings to be liberated in the presence of therapeutic touch or movement of the pelvis. Tightness here can indicate unresolved emotional tension from the past, chronic "holding on" to pain, guilt, bad feelings and/or excessive concern/enmeshment (or anti-concern/abandonment) for loved ones. Attempts to improve posture will often lead to working with emotional issues.

---

[13] Barhydt, Harrison and Elizabeth. *Self-Help for Stress and Pain*. p. 38.

To alter faulty habitual erect carriage is, in everybody's opinion, a very difficult enterprise. Especially striking is the case of persons seeking guidance of their own initiative. From the obstinate resistance encountered in such cases, it is obvious that what is attempted is really a major operation on the personality of the subject. All workers in the field agree on this point.[14]

The pelvis is associated with the Yin Principle, and the Water and Earth Elements.

30. Pelvic Lift

A back and pelvis strengthening exercise can be done from the same position. Lift up the buttocks by pushing down with the feet. In this raised position, use small differentiation movements to isolate different pelvic and lower back muscles. Then lower the back slowly, one vertebra at a time, until it rests back on the floor.

31. Pelvic Reflexes

Major pelvic reflex areas are found in the jaw, the fourth toe, the inside and outside of the heel, and the hallucis tendon on the side of the ankle. As with earlier reflex movements, we use small circular motions with the fingertips to probe a reflex area for stimulation, and both hands (one on the reflex and the other on the pelvis) for energy balancing.

For the jaw, touch the muscular areas where the jaw hinges to the skull. Feel for tension in this area. With a gentle circular motion, rub as you open and close your mouth. Make an "a-h-h-h" sound or yawn with this light or firm contact. This is similar to "energy yawns" in Paul Dennison's *Brain Gym*. A second method is a general rubbing motion, pulling down on the facial tissue all around the jaw, from the side, where the downward rubbing can be felt all the way to the

---

[14] Feldenkrais, Moshe. *Body and Mature Behavior.* p. 119.

ears, to the front. Pull the mouth open with a firm stroking motion from the lower lip to the Adam's apple area.

The fourth toe marks the water element line in the foot, the densest (most distant from the core) part of the Water Element system. Feel for tender or tense areas and use your hands to release tension by circular movement, activation or pressure. Use firm pressure to follow the tendon of the toe along the bottom of the foot.

32. Hallucis Tendon

The hallucis tendon which passes through the inner heel is an important pelvic reflex. The tendon originates at the big toe, the densest extension of the Ether energy center at the throat. The Ether center governs emotions; the hallucis is thus a way to connect Ether (emotions) and Water (attachment) zones, relating specifically to the storage of old feelings. It is an access point for old emotions stored in the pelvis. It is frequently used in bodywork for this reason.

To find the hallucis, probe with the fingers in the area just to the rear of a line between the ankle and heel. The hallucis feels like a thick guitar string, running up the inside of the leg just behind the ankle. It may be deep or shallow, so you may have to push in to find it.

This can be used with foot flexed up or down. Once you find it, push with steady pressure (light for balance, moderate or firm for change) to activate energy flow. Making sound helps dissolve the tenderness.

The hallucis has been called the "twanger," sometimes manipulated with a cross-fiber motion which feels like "twanging" a guitar chord. Done this way, the contact can be painful; this is avoided by some for

Hallucis Tendon contact point

being too forceful, and emphasized by others for the same reason. The deep Tamasic touch is most beneficial when the pressure is kept just short of the edge of resistance; pain usually indicates too much pressure.

References

Stone, R. *Polarity Therapy Vol. 1*, Book 2, pp. 20, 24, 34, 40, 75; Book 3, pp. 45-49.
Stone, R. *Polarity Therapy Vol. 2*, p. 118.
Dennison, Paul and Gail. *Brain Gym*, p. 29.

33. Butterfly Activation

This activity uses strategic placement of the legs and the activation technique to create release in the pelvic area, including the inner thigh and psoas muscles.

Method

Sit on the floor with the knees bent and the soles of the feet touching. The legs will naturally rest at the comfort level. Place the hands on the insides of the knees. Inhale and, as you exhale with pursed lips, push the legs into the hands with about 25% of your potential force.

The legs do not actually move on the push. On your inhale, as you relax, allow the legs to sink lower if they do so easily. Take up the slack with the hands. Repeat the activation from this new position. Do three times or more and then rest, allowing the body to enjoy this new position.

If desired, this can be done leaning against a wall or other back support.

Butterfly Activation

Benefits
- Lengthening of postural muscles.
- Release of tightness in the psoas and adductor muscle

groups, restoring flexibility to the inner leg/pelvic relationship.

References
Francis, John. *Polarity Self-Help Exercises*, p. 44.
Gach, Michael. *Acu-Yoga*, pp. 90 and 112.

34. Pyramid

Many teachers consider this the most artful of all Stone's "easy stretching postures." This exercise releases the hips, pelvis and shoulders, elongates the spine and opens the diaphragm. Virtually all the major pathways of energy are activated, with a simple posture that is quick and easy to do in any situation.

Method

Beginners will benefit from preparation before doing the Pyramid exercise. Possible warm-ups include psoas, hamstring and adductor lengthening exercises, pelvic or lower back reflexes and also the Butterfly Activation. Beginners can also warm up by doing portions of the posture or variations before the complete version.

To begin, stand with the feet wider apart than the width of shoulders. Lean forward, placing the palms of the hands (fingers outside, thumbs inside) on the thighs, just above the knees, and transfer the weight of the body from the legs to the shoulders. We are creating a "suspension bridge" with the arms as posts and the shoulders as cables. As you drop into the suspended position, adjust the feet a little wider to create a 90° angle at both ankle-floor and upper leg-lower leg. The knees should be directly above the ankles, and the arms and back should be

Pyramid

97

quite straight. The feet should be aligned parallel to the thighs. The shoulders should be up toward the ears. Lean forward and push the knees out with the hands to emphasize the suspension.

Once you have the posture right, experiment with gentle movement, either pulsing very lightly up and down or rocking from side to side. Then come to standing and take a moment to experience the results of the posture. You may want to do the reflexes (pelvic or shoulder) again, and then go back to the Pyramid to see if it is easier. If you are tight in the inner thighs and pelvis, use the suggested preparations. If you are unable to keep your arms straight, do the alternative Shoulder Release Pyramid on the next page.

After you are familiar with the posture, check these points for fine-tuning:
- Make sure the thighs, gluteal muscles and lower back are relaxed: the full weight of the torso should be on the hands and knees.
- Feel the spine hanging in full suspension, lengthening from its own weight.
- Make sure the back and arms are straight.
- The knees should be over the foot, and lower leg should be perpendicular to the floor.
- Each foot should be at a 45 degree angle from the center line of the body, not too wide or straight, to avoid pressure on the knees.

Pyramid in a Chair

This variation is good for older people and for those quite stiff in the pelvic area. We have used this with groups for seniors. The chair seat should be high enough to allow leg extension, so a cushion may be necessary. Sit on the chair in such a way that the legs are in the pyramid position, out to the sides with the ankles and knees making 90° angles. Place the palms of the hands on the knees (with straight arms) and gently transfer some of the weight of the torso to the shoulders. Push outward to open the pelvic area, elongate the spine, and release neck and shoulder tension. Gently rock forward and back or side to side.

Shoulder Release Pyramid

In this variation, the hands turn inward, with the fingers on the inside of the thigh. As you suspend the torso, the elbows bend and the shoulder blades are pushed toward each other in the back.

Pyramid in a Chair

This posture helps free the shoulder blades, which can become buried in tension. Rotate them forward and back, both together and alternately. You can feel the shoulder blades move and squeeze together and apart. Experiment with moving the elbows in wide circles, and pressing them toward the floor. When done, come to standing, bring the feet together, relax, breathe deeply and experience the results.

Spinal Twist Pyramid

This variation adds a twist of the spine to the normal pyramid, taking advantage of relaxation in the lower back-pelvic area and elongation of the spine to further open and energize the spinal area. This position is considered an advanced posture, so it should not be used by those who are unable to do the regular pyramid.

For the spinal twist pyramid,

Shoulder Release Pyramid

start in the regular pyramid posture. While maintaining straight arms, drop one shoulder forward. This will create a spinal twist. Turn the head to look at the floor, over the lowered shoulder, then up toward the ceiling over the upper shoulder, for further release. Make sure that the body stays in the center. Breathe and relax. Repeat the twist with the other shoulder forward.

When done, come to a relaxed standing position and feel the results. Listen to your body and use the degree of stretch and amount of time that is easy, gentle and releasing.

Leg Stretch Pyramid

This variation gives a good stretch to the back and inner portions of the thigh (adductor and hamstring muscles). Start in the regular pyramid position. Keeping the buttocks low, straighten the left leg while shifting the torso right. Make a gentle pulsing movement to lengthen the straight leg, and flex the foot at the ankle to rock back onto the heel. The pressure of the heel (a reflex to the sacrum) on the floor is beneficial for additional relaxing of the lower back. Repeat with the other leg, and alternate each side a few times. This variation can be used to take a break from having the body weight resting in the center.

Benefits
- General tension release: the Pyramid is one of the best postures for overall energy balancing.
- Because it is so quick and easy to do, even in street clothes, it is recommended for use during the day to ward off fatigue and tension.
- Stimulates circulation of cerebrospinal fluid.
- Opens the pelvic basin, allowing energy to flow up and down the legs. This is rejuvenating, good for circulation and has a grounding effect.
- Stimulating, especially due to pressure on thighs and pulsing movement.
- Relieves compression on spine.

- Stimulates shoulders (+), diaphragm (0) and pelvis (-), the three poles of the torso, unifying and amplifying energy flow and movement.
- On the level of energy theory, all systems are engaged. It is a good companion for energy balancing bodywork, accelerating energy movement in a way which would otherwise require deep contact. An excellent case history of this type of application is offered in Sills' book, referenced below.
- Excellent for pregnancy, opening the pelvic floor and toning its support muscles.

References

There are many variations for the Pyramid, and yet relatively little mention of the posture in Stone's writings. A "Pyramid-like" illustration in *Health Building* (p. 160) actually describes the Side-to-Side Ha Breath, and the reference in *Polarity Therapy Vol. 2* (p. 192) is a brief one sentence, again accompanying the Side-to-Side Ha Breath. There is a photograph of Stone in the posture in *Health Building* (p. 170), but again, there is relatively little description. An explanation is offered in the editors' footnote on page 164 of *Health Building*. The posture's popularization and development is a function of Stone's verbal classroom instruction (rather than written work), and the creativity of subsequent Polarity instructors. As its benefits were experienced, it received more attention and use, an examples of the organic, evolving nature of the art of energy-based therapies, and a validation of Stone's often-quoted motto, "Whatever works, works!"

Stone, R. *Health Building*, pp. 160, 170, 182-183.
Stone, R. *Polarity Therapy Vol. 2*, p. 192.
Francis, John. *Polarity Self-Help Exercises*, pp. 33-34.
Seidman, Maruti. *A Guide to Polarity Therapy*, p. 138.
Sills, Franklyn. *The Polarity Process*, pp. 149-152.

35. Squat

The squat is the foundation of all Stone's Easy Stretching Postures.

> After years of study of every health posture and exercise including the eighty-four Yoga postures, I have found none equal to this one which combines squatting and stretching for relaxation and well-being...
>
> What simple thing can one do to preserve bodily functions at par and stay well, or even to regain health with the expenditure of the least amount of effort and time? The answer is an easy stretching posture which is so natural that it takes only three to five minutes, once or several times a day if necessary, to increase the release of gases and the consequent intake and absorption of oxygen in the body, and to quickly release mental and emotional tension. (Stone, *Health Building*, p. 122.)

The squatting posture is a natural position assumed by much of the world's population for all kinds of daily activities. In western cultures where so much time is spent sitting in chairs and where most lives have high tension levels, many have lost the flexibility needed to do this posture. People with back problems, varicose veins and knee problems may find it difficult and possibly contraindicated. As a general rule, if there is pain anywhere, stop.

The reasons for the squat's effectiveness are explained in great detail by Stone in *Health Building*.

> ...man can take body postures which place the polarity energy fields (one immediately above the other) into action under a mild stress (or stretch) which forces them to work in two ways; first by the electromagnetic polarity; second by physical effort and gravity function, blended with the proper mental attitude. The body, the mind and the subtle energies

are therefore all engaged simultaneously. (Stone, *Health Building*, p. 111.)

Thus a primary reason for the squat's effectiveness is the close proximity of calves, thighs, solar plexus and chest, which enhances current flow in the main energy fields of the body. The squat is similar to the fetal position, creating the "path of least resistance" for energy circuits in the original weaving of the body. This position reflects the fulfillment of the involutionary energy impulse (the Yang Principle), represented by Stone's "Interlaced Triangles" geometric star, discussed on page 146.

Secondly, leveraged opening and lengthening of the pelvis and spine activates the body's natural tendency for self-correction. Just getting in this position is rejuvenating, soothing and energizing.

For many people, squatting is difficult. But it is well worth the continued effort. Stone himself could not achieve the squat position at first, but found an answer:

> The author passed his 64th birthday on February 26, 1954. He had not been able to correctly take these postures until the discovery of the gentle rocking motion to shift the polarity constantly from one group of muscles to another, which made the accomplishment of the posture possible. (Stone, *Health Building*, p. 98.)

If this posture is difficult, use movement to facilitate progress. Stone lived another 28 years after the comment above, and was pictured in the squat on many occasions, including the photos on pages 170-171 of *Health Building*, taken in the 1970s, when Stone was in his mid-eighties.

How to overcome initial difficulty? Stand with weight shifting from side to side and gradually begin the process of lowering the body down, with up and down movements. One way to help is to use a board or book under the heels (or wear shoes with heels) at first, to reduce the stretch of the calves; another is to use both sides of a door handle (see illustration, page 191) to keep balanced and support the lowering movements. We emphasize perseverance, for the benefits are well worth the effort. Specific aids for the squat found elsewhere in this book are the calf lengthening, foot flex, hamstring lengthening, scissors kick and pyramid.

Exercise instructors may consider having the class do the squat first, because of its central place in these exercises. Students will get an idea of their flexibility. All the other exercises will build toward the squat, so they can refer back to it periodically to check their progress.

> It is not the accomplishment of a position that we are after, but the stimulating actions of the currents set into motion by these posture stretches. Those who need them the most will at first feel that they accomplished the least, but they will slowly feel the benefits just the same. It is like turning on a switch and allowing the currents to do the work, instead of wasting a lot of energy in performing acrobatic stunts. All this is based on Nature's finer forces in motion. (Stone, *Health Building*, p. 139.)

Method

Stone described two squatting positions, "wide" and "narrow." He used the term "Youth Posture" for the wide position, and "Health Posture" for the narrow. They are similar in that they both require lowering the torso and resting on the haunches. In the wide position, the feet are about 12 inches or more apart, and the elbows are inside the knees, pressing out. In the narrow position, the feet are as close as possible, and the arms wrap around the legs, pressing in.

Once in the squatting position, gentle rocking will facilitate movement of energy currents and release of tension. Rocking movements can be front to back, side to side, or circular. Deep breathing, emphasizing the exhalation with a loud sigh, will also enhance the effects. After completion,

The Squat

which can mean a short or long period depending on the individual's needs and capabilities, take a resting pose, either seated on the floor, resting fully extended on the back, or standing with knees slightly bent.

To come back to standing, allow the hands to drop forward to touch the floor. Lift the back and straighten the legs, slowly uncurling to a vertical position. This "uncurling" movement is preferred over the more common vertical lift from the knees.

For therapeutic applications, Stone recommended squatting for "three minutes several times a day." (Stone, *Polarity Therapy Vol. 1*, Book 2, pages 84 and 111.)

The squat is also used in bodywork. The practitioner may assist the client in assuming the position for a short time, as a preparation or complement for other bodywork. The gravity, energy, and leverage at work in the position applies more force than the practitioner usually can create, in a more gentle way, for deeper results.

In exercise classes, the squat can be done with partners for fun and benefit. One person can stand behind the squatting student and hold the shoulders while guiding movement. Another way to work in partners is to face each other and grasp each other's wrists. Then lower each other down into the squat, each supporting the other and assisting movement.

Narrow Squat

The Health Posture has the feet about 6 inches apart at the heels, or closer. Rock into the position gently, beginning with a bend at the knees and sinking down and rising back up again. When ready to go all the way down, the hips drop toward the heels and the armpits rest on the knees. The close position of the feet gives support to the abdomen which rests on the thighs. Now begin a back and forth rocking motion.

In this position, the chest, colon and calves, the Positive, Negative and Neutral poles of the Neutral Principle, are pressed tightly together. Thus it is specifically helpful for digestion, colon function and elimination of gases.

Narrow Squat– Arms Wrapped

For this version of the Health Posture, take the narrow squat position and wrap the arms around the knees, hands locking together. This posture may be contraindicated for varicose veins. The knees are pushed together, lengthening muscles and opening the hip joints to bring spring to the step. Rock back and forth, side to side, and in a

**Narrow Squat
The "Health Posture"**

rotating motion. With locked hands, exert a gentle stretch on the arms and take a deep breath in. Exhale with a grunt or sigh, increasing relaxation. Stone's famous comment on making sound for tension relief fits well here:

> The gallant Frenchman will groan himself well while the stolid Englishman succumbs to the malady.[15]

This squat position frees the brachial plexus, moving gases and opening the heart and lung areas. It is also good for relieving constipation, toning the abdomen and thighs, and also for improving all eliminative functions. For a specific discussion, see *Health Building*, pages 134-136.

Many arm movements may be added to complement the squat. The arms may be clasped behind the back and lifted up, with the weight rocking forward to the front of the foot. The hands can be clasped behind the head, elbows lifting to open the chest. For greater lengthening, lower in the back, each hand can grasp the opposite elbow behind the head, with continued rocking from the feet. Experiment and develop your own preferences to take advantage of the squat's many benefits.

Squat with Arm Stretch

Wide Squat

The "Youth Posture" has the feet wider apart, at least 12 inches wide at the heels. The arms are placed inside the knees and the elbows exert an outward push. The hands are held firmly with interlaced fingers, a reflex shoulder release.

A balancing position can be created by placing one hand over the other in a double fist, and pressing the extended

---

[15] Stone, R. *Health Building*, p. 135.

thumbs to the eyebrows. This is the "Ridge Meets Bridge" contact shown earlier (page 34). Contact here is a reflex for the shoulders and a balancing for the Interlaced Triangles pattern (page 146). Remember to rock back and forth, side to side, in a circle, and in a twisting motion.

Many variations are possible with the Squat. The arms may be extended in back for releasing the shoulders. The feet and toes may be massaged in the position, and the Neck Lift or Neck Activation may be added. Be creative and explore the many possibilities of the Squat position.

**Wide Squat
The "Youth Posture"**

Benefits

•General enhancement of energy flow throughout the body, involving all Three Principles and Five Elements. Stone called this the "Youth Posture for Balance and Elasticity."

• Good for muscular elasticity and relaxation.
• Opens the pelvis where unexpressed emotions are stored, helping these to be released and come to consciousness.
• Relaxes the hips and perineum (especially useful in pregnancy). The latent energetic forces of the pelvis are released for rejuvenation and self-healing.
• Releases gases and stimulates the downward current of elimination.
• Eases pressure on sacrum.
• Preventative for back problems; provides a self-correcting influence for spinal tensions.

- Assists concentration and focus, centering and grounding.
- Self-nurturing; restores inner calm.
- Lengthens Achilles tendon, "unwinding" the natural stress response of the "tendon guard reflex."
- Improves colon function.

References
Stone, R. *Health Building*, pp. 98-157.
Stone, R. *Polarity Therapy Vol. 1*, Book 1, p. 49; Book 2, pp. 84-85.
Berkson, Devaki. *The Foot Book*, pp. 78-79.
Francis, John. *Polarity Self-Help Exercises*, p. 11.
Sills, Franklyn. *The Polarity Process*, p. 150.
Siegel, Alan. *Polarity Therapy*, pp. 94-96.

36. Scissors Kick

This is a gentle yet powerful exercise for opening the hip and pelvic areas. It has two effective actions for energy movement. First, the rocking of the hip joints creates expansion and contraction of the hips, which alternately puts pressure on and then releases the sacrum. This creates a pumping action that facilitates cerebrospinal fluid circulation. Second, swinging the legs enhances the transverse energy currents using the crossing-over "dynamo effect" described earlier in the Side-to-Side Ha Breath.

Because of the reflex relationship between sacrum and cranium, this type of movement of the hips leads to cranial adjustment and pressure relief. Stone recommended the Scissors Kick for relief of sinus congestion. If the nose is blocked or the head is stuffy, five to ten minutes of Scissors Kicks will often give relief.

Method

Lie face down with the head resting comfortably on crossed arms. Lift the feet so that the lower legs are perpendicular to the floor. Swing the feet rhythmically outward and inward, alternating which foot crosses in front. Some people find this easier if they emphasize the out swing, then just let the legs move on their own back to the inward position.

Repeat this easygoing motion for 5 or 10 minutes. Experiment with varying paces. Stop, lower the legs, and roll over for a period of rest. The rest period is taken on the back for a reason, because we have greater sensitivity when the sensory (front) side of the body is exposed.

As an additional energy balancing during the rest period, assume the Interlaced Triangles Balance pose (page 146), which also supports the sacrum/cranium relationship. Touch the center of the forehead with the left thumb (turning the head to the left side makes it possible to do this with the left elbow still on the floor, thus keeping the body more relaxed). At the same time, touch the pubic bone with the right thumb. These contacts balance the circuitry of the Interlaced Triangles and the sacrum/cranium reflex relationship.

Scissors Kicks can be done on the floor or on a bed. Some like to do it before rising in the morning, or to help fall asleep more easily in the evening. It can be done while reading or watching TV, and is a good supplement to weight management, hip toning (using longer times, up to twenty minutes or more daily) or back therapy programs. Both this and the following exercise are sometimes fondly called "windshield wipers." In an exercise class, this is often done at

Scissors Kick

the beginning as a warm up or at the end as a cooling down exercise.

Caution should be used for those with lower back pain or knee problems. For back protection, press the pubic bone into the floor. To protect the knees, flex the feet. If there is pain in any joint, reduce the force of the outward kick or choose a different posture to get a similar effect.

Variations

This can be done in pairs, with one person holding the left hand on the occiput and the right hand on the sacrum of the person who is doing the Scissors Kick. This is an energy balancing contact for the Yang Principle's Interlaced Triangles.

Benefits

- Good general energizer and balancer, increasing alertness. It is often used as a warm-up in exercise classes. The side to side motion benefits left/right brain integration.
- Releases lower back, especially sacrum and sacroiliac junction.
- Easy to do; good for elderly and infirm.
- Tones thighs and buttocks.
- Benefits circulation of cerebrospinal fluid, promoting mental clarity.
- Specific for sinus congestion relief.
- Releases nervousness.
- Releases tensions stored in the legs; good for "grounding" and feeling more solidly rooted in the legs and feet.

References

Stone, R. *Polarity Therapy Vol. 1*, Book 2, p. 61; Book 3, pp. 45-49.
Francis, John. *Polarity Self-Help Exercises*, p. 13.
Seidman, Maruti. *Guide to Polarity Therapy*, p.139.
Berkson, Devaki. *The Foot Book*, pp. 178-179.

37. Seated Scissors Kick

This exercise, also called Windshield Wipers, has mechanics and benefits similar to the Scissors Kick, but it can be done by those unable to do the regular posture. The rocking motion alone restores flexibility and circulation for people with limited movement capabilities.

Method

Sit on the floor (or in a chair) with the legs extended in front at a comfortably wide angle. The hands are placed flat on the floor slightly behind the body, supporting the body weight. This hand position activates wrist/pelvis reflex relationships, with additional reflex benefits coming from the pressure of the leg weight on the heel (another pelvic reflex, specifically for the sacrum).

Rock the feet rhythmically, in and out. You should be able to feel the whole leg rotating up to the hip joint. Do this for five or ten minutes. Then stop and rest, seated or lying down, experiencing the results of the exercise. The "Interlaced Triangles" contact points may be touched (left thumb to forehead, right thumb to pubic bone) as an extra balancing position.

During the rest period, close your eyes and feel the tingling sensation moving through the legs. Notice where it stops or feels blocked. You can then find an exercise to work with the blocked area. Check again later as a comparison: this exercise can be used as a gauge of energy movement in the body.

Seated Scissors Kick

Variations

This may be done leaning against a wall if the wrists are not strong or flexible enough to hold the body weight. It also may be done seated on the edge of a chair. A natural variation of this exercise can be seen when we rhythmically swing one leg as we sit in a chair with one leg crossed over the other.

Benefits
- Generates energy flow throughout the body.
- Opens pelvis and activates the cranium/sacrum energy pathway of the Yang Principle.
- Stimulates circulation.
- Side-to-side movement stimulates Neutral Principle balance, giving a sense of calm and rest.
- Good for the elderly and infirm.

38. Light Rocking Perineal

Techniques involving the perineum, or pelvic floor, are a primary foundation of Polarity Therapy.

> The perineum is the lowest major point of gravity… [and]… the major negative pole of the body... [It] holds the key to all negative and irrational impulses and perversions of the currents in the energy field. (Stone, *Polarity Therapy Vol. 2*, p. 187.)

> Perineal treatment correctly done will unlock energy blocks quicker than most other methods because it deals with the vital force of emotional locks and frustration. (Stone, *Polarity Therapy Vol. 1*, Book 2, p. 37.)

The Rocking Perineal gives an easy way to experience some of this therapeutic power. It is a natural aid to young children preparing for sleep, and first aid for emotional upset or anxiety. "The perineal contact is the best treatment for nervousness and hysteria..." (Stone, *Polarity Therapy Vol. 2*, p. 185.)

This posture connects the energy field of the pelvic floor to the upper fields of the head and shoulders; flow is increased in important autonomic nerve circuits. The gentle rocking motion stimulates energy movement and relaxation. It is similar to much-appreciated bodywork techniques taught by Milton Trager that emphasize rocking.

Method

Lie on the left side and place the left hand comfortably on the neck and the right hand on the hip, fingers reaching over the gluteal muscle and toward the pelvic floor. The little finger of the right hand should be near the coccyx. A small pillow may be used for the neck and head. Have the knees slightly bent in a position that allows stability and flexibility for rocking. When you are correctly positioned, the body will rock easily back and forth with a slight, almost-effortless movement of the upper leg. Rocking can continue for a few minutes or more.

Variations

The Light Rocking Perineal may be either done individually or in pairs. The giver of the exercise sits or kneels at the receiver's back, with right hand on the hip, fingers toward the perineum, and the left hand on the neck/shoulder junction. The giver rocks lightly, carefully being sensitive to the receiver's preferred tempo and movement. Giving and receiving a Rocking Perineal is a very nurturing experience.

Benefits

- Soothing and balancing for the nervous system. Perineal techniques are specifically recommended for the Neutral Principle's parasympathetic nervous system, governing "rest and rebuild" functions of regeneration and assimilation.
- Gives relief from nervousness or hysteria.

Light Rocking Perineal

Light Rocking
Perineal in Pairs

- Stimulates flow of energy from pelvis to shoulders and neck.
- Helpful for calming the body or soothing insomnia.
- A nice way to rock babies and children.

References
Stone, R. *Polarity Therapy Vol. 1*, Book 2, pp. 36, 37.
Stone, R. *Polarity Therapy Vol. 2*, pp. 198.

39. Foot Flex

This exercise works with the reflexes related to the sacrum and their influence in pumping cerebrospinal fluid. When walking, the rocking motion of the heel is a constant energizer. The heel itself is a reflex to the sacrum and lower back. A firm grasp of the Achilles tendon and behind the knee assists the calf muscles in lengthening; contacts on the calf itself affect colon, chest and digestive system.

Shoes play a role in energy movement: rigid soles or high heels inhibit or negate the natural therapeutic lengthening of the Achilles tendon with each step, with serious consequences for the whole body. Non-conductive rubber soles disconnect us from the earth's natural electromagnetic flow; it is healthy to occasionally touch the earth without the non-conductive barrier, such as walking barefoot in the morning dew for a few minutes.

Method

Sit comfortably with one foot crossed over the other thigh so you can easily reach anywhere on the lower leg. Find and press tender spots, pushing the thumbs firmly away from each other to encourage lengthening; the touch may be gentle or quite firm. Grasp the Achilles tendon with one hand and the calf behind the knee with the other hand. Flex the foot and hold for a count of eight. Now alternately flex and point the foot while maintaining the grasp. Do one leg and then the other. Others areas may also be touched to assist release.

**Foot
Flex**

Benefits
- Increases flexibility in the heel-calf area.
- Enhances the circulation of cerebrospinal fluid, thereby increasing mental alertness and clarity.
- Enhances ability for self expression.
- Excellent for tightness in the shins from exercise.
- Especially good for women who wear high heels, as a correction for the shortening of the Achilles tendon and lack of rocking motion. The wearing of high heel shoes is very stressful for the feet, pelvis and spine and therefore for all of the body.

References
Dennisons, *Brain Gym*, p. 19.

40. Sacral Rocking

This simple rocking motion massages the sacrum area. Through a flexing movement, the sacrum/hip area self-corrects and re-aligns itself. As the sacral area is relaxed, the spine and cranial bones may also self-adjust.

Method
Sit on the floor with the knees raised. Support your weight partially with your hands, which rest behind you.

Rock slowly and gently on the gluteal muscles in all different directions. Circles and figure eights are two good methods. The posture may also be done with partners. Standing behind the receiver, the giver gently creates and guides the movements.

Benefits
- Relief from some lower back problems, by lengthening the lower back. Reflex pressure on wrists stimulates the pelvic area.
- Relaxes hip and gluteal tension.
- Improvement of craniosacral fluid rhythm and function.
- Promotes mental clarity.

References
Mahoney, Frank. *Hypertonix*, p. 66.
Dennison, Paul and Gail. *Brain Gym*, p. 11.
Siegel, Alan. *Polarity Therapy*, p. 99.

Sacral Rocking

41. Rowing

This exercise engages several muscle systems and energy pathways simultaneously. It is grouped with pelvic exercises because its movement opens the pelvic basin and energizes the belly and lower back. The brachial plexus and shoulders, legs, lower back and pelvis and pelvic reflexes in the heels are also vigorously affected.

Rowing is stimulating and balancing for the Yang (motor and muscular) systems. The full body rocking motion eases and strengthens the back, and facilitates top to bottom balancing. Like the squat, rowing makes use of the involutionary fetal position, reflecting the compressed shape of the Yang Principle's "Interlaced Triangles" pattern (see p. 146).

The exercise has an isometric resistance between the muscles of the arms and upper back, and the legs. The degree of resistance and tempo of movement can be varied, from fast and easy to slow and hard. The upper back will be more affected with the knees bent high, and the lower back with the legs more straight.

Method

Sit with legs extended in front, knees bent. Experiment with how much to bend the knees. Reach the hands over the toes so that the palm of the hand holds the ball of the foot and the toes are pulled up and back. The fingers are thus aligned vertically with the corresponding energy lines in the feet.

Begin a motion of gentle rocking forward and back, using back muscles to pull and leg muscles to push forward. Then push forward with the feet and resist with the arms,

Rowing

letting the feet "win." Then pull back with the arms and resist with the feet, letting the arms "win." Feel the back and shoulders open and lengthen, and the pelvis flex. Keep the head low so that the neck stays relaxed.

Breathe evenly in time with the movement, exhaling forward and inhaling back. Experiment with varying tempos according to preferences and situation. The amount of time in the exercise can depend on your goals: it can be aerobic and toning if done extensively. When you are ready, stop to rest (the motor balance position, page 124, would be especially appropriate for this) and feel the results.

Variations

Increased resistance changes the dynamics of the exercise, making it a more strenuous workout for the back. By increasing the activation of the thighs, the negative pole of the Fire Element, additional stimulation of Yang energy is created. Because it is strenuous, high-resistance rowing should be done carefully, avoiding back strain.

Another variation of Rowing is done with partners. Sit opposite a partner, feet touching, both with knees bent to a comfortable degree. Join hands and take turns pulling/resisting. This can be strenuously or lightly, rapidly or slowly. Partners should be matched in general size, fitness and strength, and resistance should be sensitively applied. A class may enjoy singing "Row, row, row your boat" for fun while rowing in partners.

Another variation is combining Rowing with Toe Activation. The hands are the neutral pole and the feet the negative pole of the whole body, so the fingers and toes have a direct energy link. The fingers and toes are placed in resistance while the Rowing movement continues.

Benefits
- Opens and relaxes the pelvis.
- Exercises upper back, shoulder and chest areas.

- Good as a toning exercise for the back and legs.
- Multiple reflexology actions are used: heels (reflex to sacrum area) are pressed to the floor, fingers and toes are linked, balls of the foot (reflex to upper chest and back) are stimulated and connected with the corresponding zone of the hand.

Balancing Postures

The following postures are for quiet relaxation and rejuvenation.

> The idea presented here is that the body can be put in a [neutral] position of rest, the same as any machine. The act of standing still is anything but rest for the body. The same can be said about sitting on a chair. Even lying down has its phases of better positioning for complete motor relaxation and repair of tissues. These ideas are more or less startling until they are put to use, when we feel the difference and no further explanations are necessary. (Stone, *Polarity Therapy Vol. 2*, p. 127.)

We often use postures that give natural self-correction. Simple observation reveals many examples: resting of the forehead on the thumb and forefinger in deep thought, placing of the hands behind the skull when lying on the back, and clasping hands over the abdomen and crossing ankles while sitting. All of these commonly-assumed postures make sense from an energy anatomy perspective, unconsciously placing the energy fields in appropriate relationships for balancing. Stone's analysis of energy fields and reflexes can give meaning to what often seems to be arbitrary everyday events.

In the fast-paced modern world, much emphasis is placed on doing and achieving, and little value is placed on stillness. These postures facilitate spending some inward time to balance all the outward activity, to refresh our mental, emotional and physical resources, and to allow contemplation of inner values.

Stillness is a quality of the Neutral/Satva Principle, the subtle blueprint for the whole system. These postures usually employ a light touch to balance energy circuits.

The secret to learn here is for man's consciousness to remain still in the CENTER OF BEING, in its eternal essence. Then things will right themselves. The Holy Bible states this in simple terms: "Be still, and know that I am God."

The whole body recuperates when life's Central Energy is permitted to flow naturally, without interference by our own mind's desires, etc...

Paracelsus, the great alchemist, observed this also when he stated man is ill because he is never still. He said there was great healing in the quiet depths of space, but man never tuned into it by being quiet himself! (Stone, *Polarity Therapy Vol. 2*, p. 57.)

42. Sensory Balance Posture

In this posture the body is comfortably arranged to resemble the shape of the Yin evolutionary energy. The evolutionary attitude looks beyond material concerns in its quest for re-union with its heavenly source. Thus this posture is associated with cultivating receptivity, and is sometimes used as a meditation position.

It is also... a philosophic posture for bearing the ills of the day with a confident faith in God's Providence. (Stone, *Polarity Therapy Vol. 2*, p. 127.)

A secondary benefit is created energetically because the arms and ankles are "crossed over," affecting the Neutral Principle. It connects transverse (side-to-side) currents and inhibits any additional incoming stimulation from the outside. Thus a quality of stillness is usually experienced.

The word "Sensory" has broad implications here. Sensory and Motor are words used to summarize the functions of Yin and Yang, respectively.

Method

Sit cross-legged and rest the hands on the front of the opposite side calf area. Close the eyes and relax. At first,

Sensory
Balance

breathe consciously, with a deep inhale and exhale; then forget the breathing and rest quietly. Allow the internal energy currents to come to balance.

This can be done when sitting in a chair, either by bringing the legs up, or by extending them out and crossing at the ankles, with hands lightly clasped in front. The Sensory Balance Posture is similar to Cook's Hook-ups, p. 127.

Benefits
- Soothing, relaxing.
- Rejuvenating for the senses, especially when "overloaded." The posture integrates sensory input with mental absorption.
- Useful for meditative practices, or "getting away from it all." Helps bring the attention inward.
- Beneficial for excess or deficient Yin condition, cultivating discrimination and acceptance.
- Helps relieve the stress of exhaustion, the feeling that "we've had it up to here."

References
Stone, R. *Polarity Therapy Vol. 2*, pp. 126-127.
Francis, John. *Polarity Self-Help Exercises*, p. 45.

43. Motor Balance Posture

This position is the Yang complement to the Sensory Balance position. The pose takes the shape of the involutionary aspect of energy, the fetal position of action and involvement. The back of the head (positive pole of the motor current) is balanced with the neuter palms of the hands. The spine and back is gently lengthened. The non-crossed, straight posture affects the Yin (north-south) and Yang (back-front) Principles' energy pathways.

It is not just a position of relaxation, but rather it is also a dynamic feeling of building and potential power. Motor Balance makes sense in the context of the Yang functions of action and creativity. The posture is especially used following very active exercises like Rowing (page 117), the Ha Breath (page 70), or the Woodchopper (page 84).

Method

Sit on the floor with knees comfortably bent. Lean the elbows forward to rest on the knees and clasp the hands behind the back of the head. Breathe deeply at first, then normally. Relax and allow the energy currents to balance. Do not be concerned if the posture does not feel truly "relaxing" as it is a somewhat different state, of readiness or potential action.

Motor Balance

When we lie under a green tree and look up through its shadowy leaves, at the sky above, the motor relaxing posture ensues instinctively and automatically. We clasp our hands behind the head and cross the knees loosely. That is the life of relaxation. (Stone, *Polarity Therapy Vol. 2*, Book 5, p. 57.)

Benefits
- Relaxes, energizes before and after muscular activity
- A good complement to vigorous motor exercises like the Woodchopper and Rowing.
- Gives a gentle lengthening of spinal muscles.
- The elbow-to-knee contact is a connection of neutral (acute) and negative (chronic) diaphragm reflex points.
- Prepares the body for creativity and action.
- Balancing for front/back dimension, the Yang Principle.

References
Stone, R. *Polarity Therapy Vol. 2*, pp. 126-127.
Francis, John. *Polarity Self-Help Exercises*, p. 46.

44. Wise Man Of Old

In Stone's words, this energy balancing pose was:

...used by sages and wise men for their deeper penetration into the Inner Mysteries of life. (Stone, *Polarity Therapy Vol. 2*, Book 5, p. 57.)

Stone also calls this posture:

…the Ideal Neutral Position Squatting Posture, plus local special sense balancing through finger locations. (Stone, *Polarity Therapy Vol. 2*, Book 5, p. 57.)

It has the benefits of the squatting posture, with the addition of finger/face contacts for sensory relaxation and energy balancing for the Five Elements.

The finger contacts balance the five senses and Five Elements in the face, matching each finger with its reflexology correlate zone of the face. Thumbs in the ears relate to Ether, index fingers on the eyebrows or cheeks relates to Air, middle

Wise Man of Old
Each finger contacts an elemental zone on the face, augmenting the circuit of that element. The thumbs block the ear canals, creating an intro-spective effect.

finger at the side of the nose relates to Fire, ring finger on the lips relates to Water, and little finger on the jaw line relates to Earth.

Method

Take the squatting posture (or one of its substitutes, if squatting is not comfortable), with the elbows or armpits rest-ing on the knees, and place the fingers as noted above: thumbs in ears, first fingers.

Variations

This may be done seated in a chair and leaning forward with elbows on the knees, or with the elbows resting on the arms of the chair.

The Wise Man of Old also combines well with Hum-ming (page 165). The ear canal is blocked by the thumbs, so that the sound reverberates inside the cranium.

Benefits

• Quiets the senses. Gives a sense of introspection and inner con-templation, disengaging the mind and senses from outer stim-ulation. "The Wise Men of Old" knew that it was necessary to close off the outer senses in order to be open to the inner world.

• Balances the "vital pattern of the mind," the subtle core function of the Neutral Principle.

References
Stone, R. *Polarity Therapy Vol. 2*, pp. 56-57.
Francis, John. *Polarity Self-Help Exercises*, p. 42.

45. Cook's Hook-Ups

This posture comes from Educational Kinesiology, or Edu-K. It has two parts, which are similar to the Sensory Balance Posture (part one) and the Motor Balance Posture (part two). With both parts, a complete balance of energy currents is accomplished, involving Neutral, Yin and Yang Principles.

We do Cook's Hook-Ups whenever we feel sad, confused or angry. This cheers us up in no time.[16]

This posture was developed by therapist Wayne Cook as a way to process stimulation. It restores balance to disturbed energy circuits. Paul Dennison describes using it to counter emotional or mental stress, creating calm and release of old and new trauma.

This posture is naturally taken and commonly seen. It is often interpreted as a closed-off or resisting state of mind. However, from an energy perspective, it may be seen as taking a necessary stance for processing and digesting experience. For example, it may be used when flying on an airplane, to keep balanced in a very stimulating environment.

Method
For part one, sit comfortably with the legs crossed at the ankles. Cross the arms over the chest with hands under the position until you "feel complete," a subjective perception of stillness and becoming ready for new movement or action. Some people can feel the actual balancing taking place as tin-

[16] Dennison, Paul and Gail. *Brain Gym*. p. 31.

Cook's
Hook-ups

Part One (at left)
blocks new input
and balances.

Part Two (at
right) integrates
left and right
sides.

"Arm Position One"   "Integration Metaphor"

gles, shudders, throbs or other sensations or movements. Stay in part one until you feel this energy release: if you are very stressed, this could take some time, so be patient.

For part two, uncross the legs and arms and place the finger tips together in a "rainbow arch." Many people feel the tingling of energy crossing the fingers and balancing. This is similar to the integration metaphor part of Dennison Laterality Repatterning (page 178). Again, do this until you "feel complete."

Variations

Part one may be done in several different ways. The above posture is called a "crossover." You may also (2) "double cross" the arms and turn them under (see next page) or (3) "leg cross" while seated, with one leg over the other side's knee. Hold the ankle with one hand and the ball of the foot

Cook's Hook-ups: Variations in the Prone Position

"Arm Position Two"
Arms Double Crossed

"Integration Metaphor"

with the other hand, so that the forearms are crossed. This is a blend of the Foot Flex (page 115) and the Sensory Balance Posture (page 122). It has the added benefit of connecting the upper and lower body.

The double crossed arms position is a favorite for many. Children will challenge you to move a particular finger when the hands are clasped and turned in this way. To take the position, cross the wrists and turn the palms facing each other, then clasp the fingers. Next, turn the hands under until they rest on the chest. If this is comfortable, rest and continue. If not, use one of the other options.

Versions (1) and (2) may be done while seated, standing or lying. Version (3) is only for a seated position.

Benefits
- General relaxation and concentration. This position has proved itself in a wide variety of applications and is highly recommended.
- Release of tension. Removes distractions and allows integration of mind and emotions.
- Combines benefits of Sensory Balance and Motor Balance positions.

129

References

Cook, Wayne. *Universal Truths*, p. 132.
Dennison, Paul and Gail. *Brain Gym*, p. 31.
Stokes, Gordon and Whiteside, Daniel. *One Brain*, Ch. 8, p. 12.

46. Polarity Screens

The concept of supporting energy flow for health bene-fits started long before Polarity Therapy. Belgian inventor Leon Ernest Eeman (1889-1958)[17] suffered terrible crash injuries as a Royal Air Force pilot in WWI. Totally disabled and having no medical options, he came up with the idea of re-balancing his energy field to revive the natural polarized circuits of his body. He experienced a complete recovery, and devoted his life to the study of subtle factors underlying health.

Polarity Screens are easily made and inexpensive, or they can be purchased on the internet. Two square pieces of copper screen have copper wires attached to the corners. Rest on the screens holding a wire in each hand. For toning and general use, one wire connects the left hand (-) to a screen at the occiput or brachial plexus (+) and the other wire is held by the right hand (+) connecting it to the sacrum or feet (-). Rest on the screens for at least 5 minutes, until flow can be detected as pulsation. Reverse the polarity arrangement to reduce flow for high fever, inflammation or emotional distress.

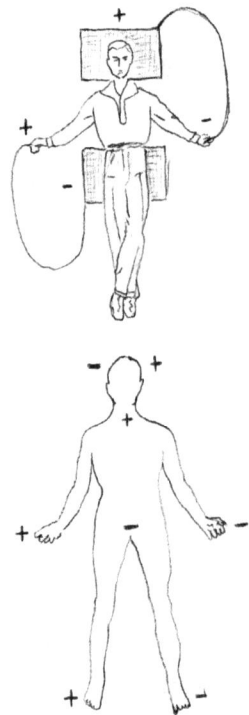

Illustrations based on Eeman; Copper wire augments biocircuits to increase energy flow.

[17] For complete information, see www.leeeman.com.

Balancing Touches

The self-help use of touch is an extension of bodywork. It can be used for stimulation, creating change, balancing or soothing. These touches can be first aid for a wide variety of stressful, painful, or difficult situations. While they are described as being self-given, all the contacts given here may also be done with two people, a giver and a receiver.

A digression on the use of hands for health is useful here. We will take a moment here to give some background on the why, how and where of therapeutic touch.

First, the point is well-made by Dr. John Thie that our modern life includes too little touching.[18] When people touch, it is usually for very limited purposes, and in extreme cases just for punishment or sex. The well-documented health benefits of touch are not appreciated or employed in many conventional health care treatments. Thus, Thie called his system "Touch for Health" to describe a distinctively new, different and good reason to touch one another.

Generally, the arms and hands resemble the jumper cables of a car battery system, with the right hand charged positively and the left hand charged negatively. This may be visualized as an outpouring fountain on the right and an incoming suction on the left.

Stone differentiated treatment into two categories, with placement of the hands determined by the situation. (Stone, *Polarity Therapy Vol.* 2, p. 208-209) He called these two types of treatment "centripetal" (from the outside in and the feet upwards) and "centrifugal" (from the head down and the inside out). Generally, centripetal treatment is for general use and stimulation, and for chronic or subnormal conditions; centrifugal is for soothing, and for acute, painful conditions.

---

[18] Thie, John. *Touch for Health.* p. 7.

In practice, the right hand is placed lower on the body (closer to the feet) than the left hand for the centripetal treatment and the left hand is placed lower than the right for the centrifugal treatment. We can visualize the effect by placing two magnets close to each other. One way has an repelling, calming effect (touching the lower or negative pole of the body with left or negatively-charged hand), the other an attracting, enhancing effect (touching the negative pole of the body with the right or positively-charged hand).

Stone emphasized the use of positive/neutral/negative poles in bodywork, and many contacts call for placement of hands according to a top-to-bottom arrangement of polarity zones (see page 27). Polarity fields are also used with a front/back (negative/positive, respectively) or left/right (negative/positive, respectively) orientation, but top/bottom orientations are more frequent in the literature, reflecting the foundational vertical axis arrangement of the spine and chakras.

Centripetal Treatment Predominates

The positive (right) hand to negative (lower) pole centripetal treatment is most frequently used.

> The operator's right hand should be on the most negative pole-- the toes, the left hand on the neuter pole, in the middle, or on the neck or head if the aroused current is strong enough to carry that far. If it is not, merely go a little above the lower contact, establish a current between the two hands by kneading and pressure, then proceed in this matter up to the neuter center pole, thence to the positive pole above that. (Stone, *Polarity Therapy Vol. 1*, Book 3, p. 40)

Understanding why this is the common placement of hands requires a larger analysis. Energy blocks occur when the impulse of cosmic force flowing through the body is disrupted or impeded by distorted pathways caused by responses to traumatic events. This can be imagined as a malfunction caused by tangled, twisted or broken wires. The result is usually a reduced capacity for current flow, experienced physically as reduced vitality or health problems, emotionally as reduced capacity for love, and mentally as reduced ability to learn and change.

Energy pathways have a dual function: conducting current down into the tissues (involution, the Yang function), and conducting a return flow back up to the mind (evolution, the Yin function). Stone emphasized the return current, the evolutionary function, as the critical focus of therapy.

> The real picture of energy block due to depolarization is given here: Wherever the negative pole of matter is in excess and rules, the positive energy field and function are crowded out. Then a shutting-in and deadlock of energies occur. (Stone, *Polarity Therapy Vol.* 2, p. 138)

Franklyn Sills' pages on this in *The Polarity Process* are excellent. This is "The Journey of the Soul," a topic explored later. Energy comes down into matter, but may become fixated and lose some of its return flow. We inevitably become attached to the forms of our minds, feelings and bodies. We gain knowledge of matter through involution (the eating of the apple in the Garden of Eden), but the ensuing attachment blocks us from moving on to knowledge of spirit through evolution.

We hold on, through the emotions of the five elements (vanity, greed, anger, attachment, fear), and the circuit is unable to be fully completed. Thus the Yin, evolutionary aspect of human experience is essential, becoming an ultimate objective for all therapies. This explains the predominance of centripetal, right-hand-below hand placement in Polarity energy balancing, as well as Stone's emphasis on perineal technique to reduce inhibitions in the five-pointed star Yin function (page 143). It also is compatible with attitude-based therapies espoused by such authors as Bernie Siegel, Louise Hay, Barbara Brennan, Norman Cousins and others.

Another way to explain the emphasis on Yin in therapy is in terms of the development of emotions. Traumas incurred in the first few years have a primary importance. In this formative period, from conception to age seven, we are very impressionable. From this period we gain most of our attitudes and expectations, and during these years emotional situations have their greatest impact. Betrayals, insults, abuses and insecurities experienced during these years set a tone for later issues and feelings.

In these formative years we are invariably occupying the Yin, receptive position in our relationships: children are powerless to resist the offenses of adults, to stop the divorce of the parents or to remove painful irritants from the environment. Such traumas set the stage for the fateful holding on described above. With early Yin experience being the source of so much later energy blockage, later Yin therapy makes sense as a primary treatment strategy.

Another aspect of Yin-oriented therapy reflects the nature of modern life. Ours is a Yang world, with constant pressure to expand and create. Meanwhile Yin qualities of receptivity and contentment are discouraged and under-appreciated. The Yin, centripetal treatment counters this tendency.

Thus the right hand below/left hand above placement is commonplace in Polarity Therapy. For many people, amplifying and facilitating the return current is a priority. The exceptions are in the instance of pain, inflammation or spasm (when the hands are reversed), and in contacts in massage or some forms of acupressure, in which hand placement is de-emphasized or considered insignificant.

Finger Polarity

On each hand, each finger has a charge; they alternate from little finger to thumb: fifth finger positive, fourth finger negative, third (middle) finger positive, forefinger negative, thumb neutral. Of the positive fingers, the middle (Fire) finger on the right hand has the strongest outgoing "push" charge, and the fourth (Water) finger on the left the greatest incoming "pull." Thus these two fingers are often used for specific applications of directional Polarity contact.

The Three Touches

As discussed before, Stone described three touches:

Quality	Terminology	Effect	Example
Light, quiet	Satva (Neutral)	Soothing, Balancing	Craniosacral
Moving, rocking	Rajas (Yang)	Stimulating	Trager
Deep	Tamas (Yin)	Penetrating	Deep tissue

Generally, the balancing Satvic touch is light and soft and used for detecting flow in the form of pulsation after Rajasic or Tamasic touches have been used. The stimulating Rajasic touch involves movement by kneading, rocking, or active other methods, and light or medium pressure. The Tamasic changing touch is firm and deep, usually without movement. Tamasic is not to be confused with excessively painful; the art of Tamasic work is to find "the edge of resistance" and wait for the client's system to invite further depth, or not. If the client is bracing in involuntary self-defense, the treatment is unlikely to have the desired effect.

All three touches are useful for practitioners, although the deep touch has been de-emphasized or deleted by some because it requires such great sensitivity. We value the Tamasic touch, with the added consideration that deep contact should be done appropriately and not in any extreme way. Stone reminds us that there is a place for deep touch in Polarity Therapy:

> A good manipulation of Polarity Centers is sometimes painful and far removed from the languid relaxation associated with magnetic treatments. (Stone, *Polarity Therapy Vol.* 1, Book 3, p. 41)

47. Tummy Rock

The Tummy Rock is one of the best known balancing touches. It works with the Yang Principle, governing digestion, circulation, action and confidence. The Yang Principle radiates in a spiraling oval, out from the umbilicus. It is the power center called the Hara in Martial Arts, the center of gravity and outgoing force. Many people can feel the radiant movement of energy from the umbilicus after the Tummy Rock, and it is often used in Polarity bodywork.

This posture has grown in popularity with use; it is minimally mentioned in Stone's written work, given as a variation of a treatment for "umbilical congestion and eye trouble." (Stone, *Polarity Therapy Vol.* 1, Book 3, chart 16)

Method

Comfortably lie, sit or stand. Place the left hand on the forehead and the right hand on the navel; the belly button can be between the thumb and forefinger. Stimulate the umbilical area by rocking the lower hand from side to side, at a tempo which feels comfortable: fast and firm will be stimulating, slow and soft will be soothing. When ready to stop, maintain the hand contact and feel energy movement as a surge, tingling or other sensation. If resting on the floor, turn the head

Tummy Rock
(also known as Jelly Roll)

to the left so that the left elbow can rest on the floor. We can feel energy movement best when completely relaxed.

Variations

This is frequently done in pairs, and often used as an introduction to the experience of energy.

A more specific use of contacts on the same points is offered by the Barhydts. The forehead is touched in the hollow above the eyebrows by thumbs and fingers, while the navel area is massaged deeply with fingertips, thumb directly in navel.

Benefits
- Balances Yang Principle and associated Yang functions.
- Stimulates and balances digestion functions; soothes upset stomachs.
- Good for building confidence.
- Frequently used to comfort young children before nap or bed-time.
- Can be used in preparation for active movement.

References

Stone, R. *Polarity Therapy Vol. 2*, p. 180.

Stone, R. *Polarity Therapy Vol. 1*, Book 2, pp. 8-11, 18; Book 3, pp. 78-79.

Barhydt, H. and E. *Self-Help for Stress and Pain*, p. 28.

Buttons

The Buttons series come from the Dennisons' *Brain Gym*. Each set of "buttons" stimulates and balances a set of acupuncture meridians based on the Chinese energy anatomy model. When the systems related to these meridians are out of balance, we feel fatigue, confusion or poor performance. When proper energy flow is restored, feelings of clarity, balance and effectiveness are regained. Each set of points is stimulated only briefly; the most time is used for holding, with a light touch. Energy moves on the basis of the contacts and does not require pressure.

The light, balancing Satvic touch used here is deceptively powerful. The movement of Rajasic touch and the penetrating, changing force of Tamasic touch are often more dramatic, but the Satvic reflects the subtlest level of energy function, the body's energetic blueprint. The Buttons series uses the Rajasic touch first to stimulate, then the Satvic touch to balance the three dualities or dimensions of brain function and energy movement: top/bottom (Earth Buttons), front/back (Space Buttons), and left/right (Brain Buttons).

48. Earth Buttons

Method

Place two fingers of one hand directly above the pubic bone and two fingers of the other hand just below the lower lip. Stimulate with the two upper fingers and then gently hold both contacts. Breathe deeply, visualizing the movement of energy up the center of the body. Add looking up and down with your eyes (without moving the head) to assist the top-bottom connection. When "complete," remove the hands from their contacts. Repeat with the opposite hand holding the points. Finish by looking all around in a downward direction: downward eye placement activates the brain's top/bottom dimension. This emphasizes the feeling of being grounded and anchors in a feeling of being grounded.

Benefits
- Helps to restore energy flow in the Central (or "Conception") Meridian which comes up the center of the body on the front starting directly above the pubic bone and ending below the lip. This corresponds to the Yin Principle and the Earth Element in Polarity.
- Integrates top/bottom dimensions, for "grounding" or feeling more stable and practical.
- Good for activities like mathematical calculations or balancing a checkbook.

Reference
Dennison, Paul and Gail. *Brain Gym*, p. 26.

Earth Buttons

49. Space Buttons
Method

Place two fingers of one hand at the junction between the coccyx and the sacrum, the hard boney area at the base of the lower back. Place two fingers of the other hand on the "mustache area," between the upper lip and nose. Stimulate with the two upper fingers and then hold. Breathe deeply, and imagine a movement of energy up the back and over the top of the head to the upper lip. You may experience energy movement and balance. Stop when you feel complete.

Space Buttons

Repeat with the opposite hand holding the points. Finish by looking all around in an upward direction. This emphasizes the upward direction and anchors a feeling of the expansiveness of space.

Benefits

•Helps restore proper energy flow to the Governing Meridian which comes up the center of the body from the tail bone over the head to directly above the upper lip. This corresponds to the Yang Principle in Polarity.

•Helps with back-front brain integration, controlling such activities as quick decision making.

Reference

Dennison, Paul and Gail. *Brain Gym*, p. 28.

50. Brain Buttons

Method

Place one hand so that it covers the navel. This is a linking point for all the acupuncture meridians. With the other hand, touch on either side of the sternum just under the clavicle (collar bone). In acupuncture, these points are the top of the kidney meridian, called K27. Use two fingers to contact one side and the thumb to contact the other. Rub with the upper hand to stimulate and then stop and hold. Move the eyes left and right, crossing the midline, as an optional extra stimulation. Stop when you feel complete.

Benefits
- Integrates left and right brains.
- Restores energy flow in the kidney meridian. This corresponds to the Neutral Principle in Polarity.
- Facilitates activities that require total brain function such as reading or using eyes in concentrated study.
- Opens the mental perspective when you feel overly focused on details or "one-sided" on an issue. Helps make both sides visible.

Reference
Dennison, Paul and Gail. *Brain Gym*. p. 25.

51. Brain Energy Balance

This is a quick and simple meridian balance, combining the three preceding poses.

Method

In all three parts, hold one hand so that the fingertips surround the navel. For right/left balance, stimulate and hold the same acupuncture points as brain buttons, on each side of the sternum, called K27. For top/bottom balance, stimulate and hold with the thumb below the lower lip and two fingers above the upper lip. For back/front balance, stimulate and hold directly behind the navel on the back. Stop each section when it feels complete.

Brain Buttons

Benefits
- Balance of the top-bottom, left-right, back-front dimensions of energy flow and brain function.

Reference
Barhydt, H. and E. *Self-Help for Stress and Pain*, p. 19.

52. Balance Buttons
Method

Place one hand with the fingertips covering the navel. With two fingers of the other hand, contact the indentation at the base of the skull about one inch behind the ear. Combine deep breathing with visualizing the movement of energy up from the navel to the head, holding for a minute or so. Do one side, then switch hands and do the other. Sense the effect on the body and stop when you feel complete.

Benefits
- Links the navel with points affecting balance, creating a state of relaxed body, alert mind.
- A good stress release break for computer workers.

Reference
Dennisons, Paul and Gail. *Brain Gym*, p. 27.

53. Positive Points

These contacts are called "Positive Points" in Brain Gym and "Stress Release Points" in Touch for Health. The position and effect is similar to Stone's Wise Man of Old (Page 125).

Holding this area of the forehead helps to process emotional stress from past and present. These are reflex points for emotional centers of the brain.

Positive Points are useful to calm a stressful emotional response, or to help process an emotional memory. The contact is also used for soothing another person, such as a child who is upset or during an emotional release accompanying bodywork.

Method

Contact the forehead lightly on both sides, just above the eyebrow and midway between the hairline and brow. Use either both hands, two fingers on each side, or one hand, thumb on one side and two fingers on the other. A slight bulge, the frontal eminence, is the exact location. Hold this gentle contact until you feel complete.

Benefits
- Ability to approach goals with less worry and emotion.
- Makes it easier to face situations that have been upsetting.
- Diffuses emotional tension.

References
Thie, John. *Touch for Health*, p. 36.
Dennison, Paul and Gail. *Brain Gym*, p. 32.
Stone, R. *Polarity Therapy Vol. 1*, Book 2, p. 52.
Barhydt, Harrison and Elizabeth. *Self-Help for Stress and Pain*, p. 16.

Interlaced Triangles & Five-Pointed Star

The next poses create balance in two basic circuits of the energy anatomy. The Interlaced Triangles (or Six-Pointed Star) and the Five-Pointed Star are two of the most frequently used maps in Polarity Therapy. These geometric shapes track wireless circuits which have a major significance in all three principles and all five elements.

The Interlaced Triangles pattern is the basic template for manifestation, including humanness. In three dimensions, it is represented by the star tetrahedron, greatly valued in sacred geometry and Hermetic Philosophy, both important sources for Stone's work. This pattern precedes the formation of the body itself, and represents the creative impulse of Spirit as it begins movement into Form.

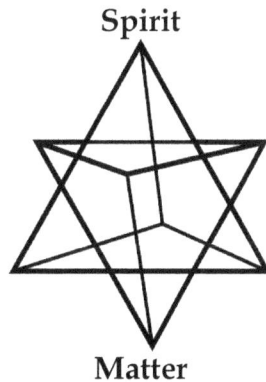

Spirit

Matter

Due to its association with the creative, initiating impulse, the Interlaced Triangle pattern is associated with, but not the same as, the Yang Principle. The actual Yang energy pattern is found in the Umbilical Spiral current and in back-front relationships. The

Interlaced Triangles
(also known as the Six-Pointed Star)

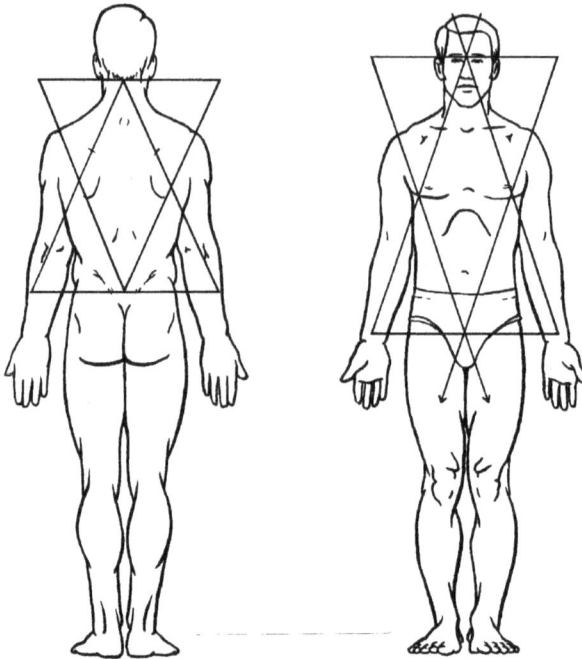

two triangles represent the downward-pointing Yang incarnation and materialization experience, and the upward-pointing Yin evolutionary and spiritualization experience, both essential for the purpose of life. The triangles are identifiable in the body in the triangular shapes of the occiput, sacrum and heel, all highly valued for energy balancing hand positions.

As the Interlaced Triangle pattern represents the impulse to create, the Five-Pointed Star pattern represents the result of that impulse, the human body. The Five-Pointed Star is the fulfillment of the downward, creative, materialistic impulse and the platform for the upward, spiritualistic Return to Source.

The Five-Pointed Star is associated with the Yin energy, but it is not the same. The actual Yin energy pattern is found in Long Line current flow circuits and in bottom-top relation-

Five-Pointed Star
Pattern

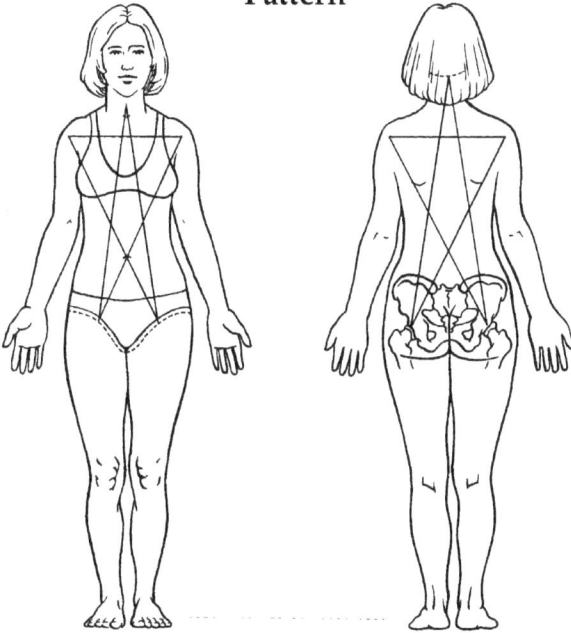

ships. A substantial portion of Polarity Therapy bodywork involves the Five-Pointed Star in some form, to support the recovery from materialistic fixation and a return to spirit.

In Traditional Chinese Medicine the shape of the Interlaced Triangles is considered significant in body characteristics of gender.[19] The downward pointing energy of the Yang triangle is reflected in broader shoulders, downward pointing beard, and protruding sexual organs of the male. The upward moving energy of the Yin triangle is reflected in a female's broader hips, higher voice, indented sexual organs, and other characteristics. Both man and woman have both triangles

[19] Kushi, Michio. *The Book of Macrobiotics.* pp. 86-87, 9. Also see Muramoto, *Healing Ourselves.* pp. 8-9, 21-37. Sources from East Asia are strong in describing Yin and Yang characteristics in all aspects of life. Integrating East Asian and Polarity energy models is discussed later, on page 253.

(and both stars), with the impact of one slightly predominating according to gender.

Exercises for the Interlaced Triangles have an inward (flexion) shape, such as found in the Squat. This mirrors the fetal position, in which the body materialized as it became "involved" (involution) in the world. This pose exposes the back Yang side and protects the front Yin side. The top and bottom points of the triangles are emphasized.

Five-Pointed Star exercises have an outward (extension) shape, such as found in the Taoist Arch. These mirror Yin's quest for meaning beyond materialism (evolution). There is significance in all five outer points (hips, shoulders and throat), plus all five inner points (umbilicus, each side of the diaphragm and each K27 point on each side of the sternum below the clavicles) that create a pentagon. In addition the actual lines connecting the points hold reflexes for virtually all of the body's organs and systems.

Many exercises deliberately go from one pattern to the other: the Woodchopper and Rocking Cliff are examples. These embody a smooth, balancing, pendulum-like flow from Yang to Yin and back.

54. Interlaced Triangles Balance

The Interlaced Triangles points and contacts are more subtle than the Five Pointed Star, and only two of its points are actually in the physical body. In the front, the two points in the body are the "Third Eye" at the top, and the pubic bone at the bottom; thus the pattern reflects a relationship between Apollonian consciousness at the top and Dionysian unconsciousness in the pelvis; it is important for these two poles to be able to function in a balanced, coordinated way.

In the back, the Interlaced Star pattern is associated with the powerful structural relationship between cranium and sacrum; when one is disturbed and not level, the other tends to compensate. Polarity Therapy and Craniosacral Therapy

Interlaced Triangles Balance
Connect the top and bottom points and wait
for pulsation to become palpable.

both emphasize major therapeutic opportunities at these locations. In advanced methods, subtle factors relating to these bones' positioning and pulsation receive primary attention.

Method

The balance involves holding the top and bottom points of the star. Experiment with left and right hands above and below, to determine the best placement. Thumbs are often used, but any comfortable contact is acceptable. The points of the star are forehead to pubic bone in front, occiput to sacrum in back. A same-side connection of shoulders to hips can also be used, but the top and bottom points are the primary focus. Lying down is most relaxed, but these contacts may be made in any position. It is easy to do seated in a chair.

Benefits
- Balances the Yang Principle, enhancing responsibility and creativity.
- Helpful in correcting imbalances between conscious and unconscious aspects of self. For example, when wanting to bring consciousness to an unconscious emotional or sexual tendency.
- Balances the back, motor current side of the body.
- Soothes the central nervous system.
- Relaxing for feelings relating to authority, forcefulness, confidence and action.
- Assists movement of cerebrospinal fluid.
- Complements bodywork or exercise for the back.

Reference
Stone, R. *Polarity Therapy Vol. 1*, Book 2, p. 18.

55. Five-Pointed Star Balance

The pelvis and throat are highlighted by this balancing contact. The pelvis is the storage vault for feelings, the reactions to earlier stimulation. In this contact, the pelvis is linked by the arms to the throat, where feelings are verbalized. Feelings must be able to be expressed, or they become emotionally toxic to the energy systems.

Five-Pointed Star contacts are especially significant in emotional processing. They are also used for improving abdominal and thoracic organ functions, like digestion and breathing, and for facilitating expression of feelings. They are commonly used when working with eliminative functions including the colon. Since back problems often originate in front tension, the Five-Pointed Star is also commonly used with structural balancing of the spine, hips and shoulders.

Method

For the Five-Pointed Star contact, lie comfortably on the floor or bed. Touch the left pelvic area with the right palm, and the right upper chest area (fingertips touching the shoulder) with the left hand. Hold this position until you feel complete, which may be experienced as tingling, softening, heat or pulsation, followed by a quietness or settled feeling.

Next, move the upper hand to rest gently in the throat area (approximately at the "Adam's apple"), making a con-

Five-Pointed Star Balance
Connect the five points and wait for pulsation to become palpable.

tact at the top of the five pointed star. Now the link is between the pelvic area and the throat. Again wait for the energy to release and balance.

Next do the same contacts to the right pelvic area with the left hand and the left shoulder with the right hand and then move the upper hand to the throat. Be conscious of the energy movement and when you feel complete, take a moment to relax and experience the new balance.

A "butterfly" variation is shown in the illustration. Lie on the back with the knees bent and the soles of the feet touching, knees widely open. Let the weight of the legs gently open the pelvis as the five pointed star contacts are made.

Benefits
- Balances the Yin Principle, enhancing receptivity and contentment.
- Opens and lengthens pelvic muscles.
- Helpful in emotional release and balance.
- Provides a complementary postural balance following exercises for the back, as it opens and balances the front of the body.
- Beneficial for visceral function of any organ.

Reference
Stone, R. *Polarity Therapy Vol. 1*, Book 2, p. 16.

56. Bridge Reflex

These points relate to the junction of neck and shoulders. When this area of the body is blocked, the brachial nerve plexus is inhibited and breathing and relaxation suffer. These points are also used to release eye tension.

Method

Take a position in which the head can rest on the hands: squatting is best, or seated at a table. Place the curled fist of one hand inside the other, leaving the thumbs extending out and next to each other. Use these two thumbs to contact the area just to the side of where the bridge of the nose and the ridge above the eye meet (these spots may be tender). Maintain the thumb contact. Pressure or a circular motion here may assist in release.

Benefits
• Helps to restore balance in breathing and movement of gas.
• Balances side-to-side Neutral Principle.
• Good to counteract dizziness after exercise.
• Releases shoulder-neck tension and allows the circulation to balance between the head and the rest of the body.

References
Stone, R. *Polarity Therapy Vol. 1*, Book 2, p. 85.

57. Sympathetic ANS Reflexology Session

This combination of contacts comes from an advanced Polarity Therapy technique. It is mainly for use in a Polarity session, with a giver and a receiver. However some of the benefits are also available for the individual using just the part of the technique which can be done alone. Although it is not primarily a self-help method, it is included partly because it is not described in other Polarity Therapy literature.

Writing long before the discovery of the Social Engagement system (also known as the Polyvagal Theory[20]) in the 1990s, Stone considered the sympathetic branch of the autonomic nervous system (ANS) to be the Yang subdivision of the overall nervous system. He considered the Parasympathetic ANS to reflect the Neutral Principle and Cerebrospinal (voluntary, somatic) system to reflect the Yin Principle. These allocations have been the subject of some discussion, not least because of inconsistencies in Stone's language; he was far ahead of his time and used old-fashioned terms that are occasionally not easy to interpret.

---

[20] See www.energyschool.com for resources to understand the Polyvagal Theory. Assuming that triune functionality is present in any system, the nervous system could be viewed as neuronal/glial/CSF, limbic/reptilian/neocortex, sympathetic/parasympathetic/social, central/ANS/fascia, and other three-part conceptualizations.

Sympathetic ANS Reflexology Session,
Step by Step Touch Sequence

1. Find the sorest cervical segment.

2. On the Table on p. 153, look up which other vertebrae correspond to the sorest cervical.

3. Start at the foot and work up, pressing and holding approximate reflex points in the triad.

C1
C6
T9
T12
L5

L5
T12
T5
T1
C7
C1

L5
L3
L2
T12
T6
T1
C1

Use this chart to locate reflexes according to the "Chart of Spinal Relationships" on the next page.

The primary function of the sympathetic ANS is mobilization for normal needs. Its stress response is the "fight or flight" response. The point has been well made by Pelletier (see page 246) and others that modern life often affords neither fight nor flight as a realistic option. Thus the sympathetic system can be on all the time, leading to chronic anxiety followed by exhaustion, eventually leading to depression and parasympathetic de-mobilization. Often chemical treatments (sedatives, sleeping pills, blood pressure regulators, intoxicants) are used to artificially give relief from chronic sympathetic nervous system overload, but these have many significant disadvantages

This balance can relieve the sympathetic ANS fight or flight pressure. It is based on the reflex relationships between spinal vertebrae and their reflexes in the feet and legs.

Method

Lie down on the floor or bed, or recline in such a way that the weight of the head is entirely supported and the neck is relaxed. With the fingers touch the sides of the neck firmly to determine which side and which vertebral spinous processes (the bone projecting from the sides of the spine) are the most tender and painful to the touch.

Start at the head behind the ears, and touch firmly on each side of the neck, in steps going down. Estimate which vertebra is most sore and find it in the left column in the chart. Then look next to that vertebra, in the center and right columns, for the lower related vertebrae. Then use the drawing to figure out where the reflexes to these vertebrae are, on the feet and in the leg. The full treatment in an advanced Polarity session makes progressive contacts starting at the foot, touching each reflex firmly, and ending at the top in the neck where we started. In all contacts a firm touch is used initially, then a light touch is held until pulsation is detected and synchronized between any two points.

For the self-given version, we touch only the foot and leg. Using the chart to approximate the right location, press deeply on the inside edge (the Ether line) of the foot. The right hand starts near the toe, the other in the arch. The right spot will be painful to the touch.

Feel for a release of these points, then move on. Now the hand that was at the toe moves up to replace the hand near the arch, which in turn finds the next spot, inside the heel.

Chart of Spinal Relationships		
(+)	**0**	**(–)**
C1	T3	L5
C2	T4	L4
C3	T5	L3
C4	T6	L2
C5	T7	L1
C6	T8	T12
C7	T9	T11
T1	T2	T10

The vertebrae are linked in triads from their origin in the early embryo. Find the sorest vertebra from the column on the left, and then make matching contacts from the center and right columns. This can release the sympathetic branch of the autonomic nervous system. Start with reflexes in the foot, then the contacts in the leg, and then connect the point in the back.
Reference: Beaulieu, John. *Polarity Workbook*. p. 183.

Again, press firmly until you feel energy release as a pulse, tingling or relaxation.

Next, move up again. The lower hand assumes the position at the heel, while the upper hand finds the next spot near the Achilles tendon on the outside of the leg behind the heel. After a time, the upper hand moves up again to the next place in the calf, on the rear outside below the knee, then finally to the top leg position in the thigh.

After the sequence is complete, go back to the spot on the neck that was sore. Very often the pain will now have melted away!

Benefits
- Good for stress, sleeplessness, agitation, exhaustion, anger, or fearful conditions.
- Combines well with the Light Rocking Perineal (page 113).
- Gives a sense of centered balance and calm power.

References
Stone, R. *Polarity Therapy Vol. 2.* pp. 85-91, 163-165, 197.
Beaulieu, John. *Polarity Therapy Workbook.* p. 183.

58. Path of Fire

A primary Polarity Therapy circuit for Yang is the "Path of Fire," in which the first knuckle of the second toe is stimulated with a firm (Tamasic) touch, then balanced with a light touch. This posture is an adaptation of the familiar General Session contact, to create a self-help approach.

Method

Sitting in the Sensory Balance position, hold the second toe with thumb and forefinger on both sides. Squeeze both for a minute, then shift to a light (Satvic) touch and wait for pulsation to be detected at the point of contact. The firm phase can be supplemented with moving (Rajasic) touch, such as pulling, rocking and squeeze-release. The full elapsed time could be five minutes of alternating touches, always ending with the light touch.

This exercise supports Yang energy including outgoing expression, will power, determination, decisiveness and muscular strength. Because Yang and Yin are interdependent, this pose also can be calming and restorative. In addition, the Path of Fire is a circuit connecting important digestive points and reflexes. Use this contact for digestive support of any kind, especially liver, gall bladder, stomach and duodenum. It is also useful for relief from headaches and eye problems, especially in the frontal/orbital area, including the sinuses.

Students occasionally ask why the second toe is used for the Path of Fire, when fire (as in Fire Element) normally refers

Path of Fire Balance

The contact is on the knuckle of the second toe, using firm contact initially. Wait for a sense of pulsation and flow, and lighten the touch as the pulsation synchronizes and amplifies.

NL

to the third digit on the hands and feet. The answer requires differentiation between the Three Principles and the Five Elements.

Dividing the foot longitudinally into three zones, the middle section represents the Yang Principle (+), with Neutral (0) as the more medial and Yin (-) as the more lateral sectors. The first knuckle on the second toe represents the most distal (furthest from the core) contact in the Yang sector of the foot. The most distal point on any circuit is where that energy is most densely coalesced.

Differentiation between Principles and Elements is a hurdle for every Polarity Therapy student. Stone did not make this easy: in his books, written over many years, the term Fire is used for both Yang Principle and Fire Element. Similarly he refers to Water for both Yin Principle and Water

Elemental references and Air is used to discuss both Neutral Principle and Air Element. The intended meaning can be derived from the context.

Benefits
- Stimulates Yang energy for more power, heat and commitment.
- Helpful for problems with digestion, eyesight and nervousness.
- Sometimes helpful for headaches and sinus problems.

References
Stone, R. *Polarity Therapy Vol. 1*, Book 3. Charts 7, 8.
Sills, Franklyn. *The Polarity Process.* p. 111.

Related Exercises
Interlaced Triangles Balance (Six-Pointed Star) (p. 146).
Tummy Rock, also known as Jelly Roll (p. 136).
Rowing (p. 117).

59. Ear Reflexes & Thinking Cap

The ears are microcosmic representations of the whole body; ear acupuncture is a sophisticated specialty in Traditional Chinese Medicine. The ear shape reflects the shape of the fetus in the womb: shoulders at the top, pelvis below, with the ear canal relating to the umbilicus. The customs of puncturing the earlobe (a pelvic reflex) at puberty, and wearing gold (a stimulant) can be interpreted as subconscious energy adjustments for water chakra stimulation.

Stone considered the ear lobe to be an indicator of vitality, the positive pole (wrist bracelet being neutral and buttocks being negative poles) indicator of vital force or reserve energy. The amount of this vitality is not just inherited genetically,

Three Zones of the Foot

The first knuckle of the second toe is the most distal point of the Yang Zone, when subdividing the foot longitudinally. This gives a rationale for the Path of Fire terminus being at that point.

Ear Reflexes

Contact on the ear will stimulate energy movement in the
corresponding area. All three
touches (light, firm and moving) can be used, but end
with a light touch to sense
pulsation, indicating flow.

it is also a reflection of the diet, lifestyle and emotions of parents and previous generations.

Method

Sit, squat, or lie down comfortably. The fingertips are
placed in the ear canals with light pressure, light movement
or soft touch. In addition, pulling and twisting the ear in all
directions activates reflex relationships to the whole body.

Variation

In Educational Kinesiology, the "Thinking Cap" is used
to improve concentration and comprehension. It consists of
rolling and unrolling the ears, repeated three or more times.

Benefits
• Affects sense of sound, relating to the Ether Element and the
  central core of the body. Combines well with making sound for
  refreshed concentration and calm.
• Gives a general reflexology treatment for the whole body.
• Firm contact on the ear canal in four main directions (up/
  down, back/front) is a release for Yang motor tension.
• Enhances balance and digestive functions of the umbilical area.
• Feels great as part of a massage or bodywork treatment, espe-
  cially as part of a scalp rub.

References
Stone, R. *Polarity Therapy Vol. 1*, Book 2, p. 79.
Stone, R. *Health Building*, pp. 150-153.
Francis, John. *Polarity Self-Help Exercises*, p. 16.
Thie, John. *Touch for Health*, p. 120.

60. Tennis Ball Head Cradle (Stillpoint Induction)

This simple procedure induces self-correction. By lying with the back of the head head resting on two tennis balls, putting pressure on the occiput, we can induce what is called a "stillpoint," which Upledger defines as:

> ...a therapeutic interruption of craniosacral rhythm which allows the craniosacral system to reorganize its activity for more optimal effect on the body.[21]

The craniosacral system is the central core of the body including the spine, cranium and sacral area. Polarity Therapy has several maneuvers for cradling the head (Stone, *Polarity Therapy Vol. 2*, p. 139) and Stone knew about the cranial techniques that were just emerging in his era:

> Polarity current research in cerebrospinal fluid and in craniopathy: The life-breath or Prana current moves in the cerebrospinal fluid conductor to all tissue cells and communicates with other internal secretions and body fluids, like a living cosmic breath. This may be called the primary respiratory cycle of energy flow, with its own cranial rhythmic impulses as a physiological wireless energy response, like atomic current circuits. It is prior to and distinct from the regular respiration of the lungs' cycle of oxidation and pulse beat. (Stone, *Polarity Therapy Vol. 2*. p. 223)

Method

This exercise requires a prop, two tennis balls bound closely together or a rubber device made for the purpose. The tennis balls are tied snugly in a sock or connected and tied together with string through holes. They must be bound so that the balls stay together. The Energy Exercises classroom can have these available for use.

---

[21] Upledger, John. *Craniosacral Therapy*. p. 238.

Take the "tandem tennis balls" and place them under the head so its full weight rests on them, one ball on each side of center, about midway up the back of the skull. The specific location can be located by finding the boney occipital prominence at the base of the skull and feeling above it for a slight depression.

Rest the head on the tennis balls for about 10 minutes or a length of time that feels good. If needed, adjust the head slightly, with gradual, gentle movement, to maintain comfort. If pain arises in any form, it is time to stop.

Variations

Curl the hands into fists and let the head rest on the knuckles as you rest on the floor or bed. This will not work if shoulder tension is created by having the arms raised during the posture.

Benefits
- Adjustment of the craniosacral system.
- Reduces stress, enhances body function, relaxes connective tissue, enhances fluid motion and reduces fever.
- Can be effective for headache relief.
- Has been used with people with auto-immune disease, autism in children, degenerative arthritis and anxiety.

References
Upledger, John. *CranioSacral Therapy*, pp. 310-311.
Stone, R. *Polarity Therapy Vol. 1*, Book 2, p. 49, Book 3, pp. 48, 79, 101.
Stone, R. *Polarity Therapy Vol. 2*. pp. 45, 162.
Gach, Michael. *Acu-Yoga*, p. 117, also pp. 173-174.

Stillpoint Induction

Pressure on each side of the occiput, behind the ears, influences the body's natural rhythm of expansion and contraction, with benefits relating to increasing mental and physical vitality.

JC

61. Fountain Of Love

This exercise was practiced by famed Montessori educator Elizabeth Caspari (1899-2002),[22] who taught at the Polarity Center at Murrieta Hot Springs CA in the 1980s.

Method

There are eight "sets" in the routine, for hands, arms, chest, shoulders, head, torso, legs and finishing. Dr. Caspari suggested doing them while singing, humming or whistling; she sang the following words from her Mazdaznan ("Master Thought," a Persian mystic tradition) song book.

> Fountain of Love, Our source is in thee.
> Living thy will, the spirit is free
> O Beautiful day, When all of us see
> The hope of the world is Love

Shake the hands up and down, loosely held in front of the chest, palms facing the chest. Shake the hands up and down with palms facing downward, elbows bent, arms relaxed, fingertips straight ahead. Make a parcel: roll the arms hand over hand away from the body, then do the same toward the body.

Arms: Reach the arms up and out one at a time, shaking the hands as you reach the limit. Repeat doing both hands together. With a loose hand tap one arm, rotating it to reach all surfaces. Do the same with the other arm.

Hold arms extended in front, palms up. Put the hand into a fist with thumb extended, and press gently into the armpit area. Move the elbows out to the side and back, pressing in with the thumbs.

Shoulders: Roll the shoulders forward and backward in circles as if touching the ears.

Head: Sing with a "La-la-la-la" to the roof of the mouth (it is difficult to sing words while moving the head, and this

---

[22] For info, see www.caspari-montessori.com/history/.

also stimulates reflexes in the roof of the mouth). Nod the head forward, then rotate left and right. Keep the shoulders down and the head up.

Circle forward circles, then backward circles, with the chin. Then make figure eights with the chin, first one way, then the other. Lean the head over so the ear "listens to the sky," in both directions.

Lightly tap the head all over with the fingertips going all the way down to the shoulders.

Torso: Tap the chest all over strongly with the fists. Embrace yourself with both arms and lean forward, lengthening the back. Do this leaning forward to the left and then the right. Then, use your fingertips to tap lightly going down to the shoulders.

Legs: Lying on the back or seated in a chair, lift one knee, then the other as if marching then lift both knees. Move the toes with legs straight, one foot at a time, then both at once. Circle feet one way, then the other. Shake feet one at a time, then both together.

Finish: Standing up, tap the legs with the side of the hands. Begin at the feet and go up to the side of the hips. Tap the front, sides and back of the legs and buttocks.

Reach the hands up to the left and then the right, fully extending the arms and shaking the hands and sending love to the world.

Stand quietly and feel your body and how it has both come alive and relaxed.

Benefits

- Caspari attributed her vitality (traveling worldwide teaching the Montessori Method in her eighties) to this exercise set. She was 103 when she died.
- Gives a feeling of well-being and joy.

62. Thymus Thump

The controller of energy flow in the body is the thymus gland... The thymus gland is the first organ to be affected at an energy level by an emotional state.[23]

Method

Use the fingertips to lightly tap the center of the upper chest area. For a more vigorous stimulation, make fists and rap more firmly with the knuckles, like Tarzan. If the setting is right, add a Tarzan yell for extra invigoration.

Benefits

• Increases overall vitality.
• Gives a sense of openness to love.
• Beneficial for the heart and immune system.

Reference

Diamond, *Your Body Doesn't Lie*, pp. 53, 67.

---

[23] Diamond, John. *Your Body Doesn't Lie*. p. 61, 83.

Balancing Sounds

Audible sounds reflect an essential form of energy.

...the fundamental level of the whole world, according to the Vedic rishis, is made of sounds.[24]

The Biblical phrase has an esoteric meaning: "In the beginning was the Word, and the Word was with God and the Word was God." Mystic Eastern philosophies describe a cosmic emanation of sound and light which precedes all phenomena. The ability to perceive this celestial emanation with inner senses is a theme of spirituality in many traditions.

Music

Music can be a powerful tool in healing strategies. Music has the power to transform feelings, evoke expression, and inspire change. In *Music and Sound in the Healing* Arts, John Beaulieu cites research in which patients exposed to music healed more quickly than patients in control groups. Different kinds of music have different effects, and the effects may be highly individual according to each person's subjective perspective. Beaulieu gives general guidelines for analyzing sounds according to the elements, using rhythm, speed, volume, pitch and key. The slower and lower the sound, the lower the related energy center. Beaulieu links keys to the Five Elements as follows:

C (256 cps)	Earth
D	Water
E	Descending Fire
F	Descending Air
G	Ascending Air
A	Ascending Fire
B	Ascending Water
C (512 cps)	Ether[25]

---

[24] Chopra, Deepak. *Quantum Healing.* p. 250.

[25] Beaulieu, John. *Music and Sound in the Healing Arts.* pp. 95-96.

Yehudi Menuhin summarizes the value of music in his foreword to Patricia Joudry's *Sound Therapy for the Walkman*:

> Music is the voice of the universe, it is the voice of humanity and is part of our existence. Good music is the harmonization of all the vibrations of which matter consists, and it restores us to ourselves and to our universe. It is the bond that we have between our frequencies and those frequencies which vibrate millions of light years away.
>
> When we hear music we are actually vibrating with the whole audience, and with the performer, and we are thereby put in touch with the composer's mind and heart.
>
> I have always felt that music is basically therapeutic, restoring proportions which are squeezed out of shape by the pressures of the day. In a state of physical disequilibrium of the nerves or the mind, music can reach our subconscious and put things in place.[26]

There are two sides of the sound therapy equation, as Beaulieu points out: changing the music, and changing the listener. For the first, we can actively cause certain types of music to occur, by playing selected sounds, or experimenting with tuning forks or other instruments. The possibilities for doing this, such as playing selected music for specific purposes, singing various kinds of songs, etc., are innumerable.

On the other hand, we can experiment with the receptive approach and develop a consciousness which perceives all sound as music, attuning ourselves to harmonize with the natural sounds of our local environment.

> During listening you have the power to resonate with your sonic environment. Suspend your mental attitudes, relax, and open yourself to the energy of

---

[26] Joudry, Patricia. *Sound Therapy for the Walkman*. p. vii.

sounds. The deeper the relaxed listening, the more there is to be discovered.[27]

This novel concept mirrors Stone's emphasis on the Yin or evolutionary aspect of energy as a primary focus of therapy. In this receptive listening, we seek greater flexibility, receiving openly and responding spontaneously, instead of following rigid preconceptions. These are the attributes of a healing process for the evolutionary aspect of energy.

63. Humming

> Humming in high and low pitch can be used selectively to vibrate any area of the head or body where the hands are placed for polarization. (Stone, *Health Building*. p. 111)

Humming uses the skull and abdomen to act like the hollow sounding board of a guitar or similar musical instrument. The relationship between types of sound and energy centers can be explained in scientific terms:

> In the case of sound, for example, the air in a cavity will respond only weakly to a sound wave coming from outside, but will begin to 'resonate,' or vibrate very strongly, when the sound wave reaches a certain frequency called the resonance frequency.[28]

Each sound has a vibration of its own and can be used to create vibration in a selected body area. Low pitched sounds resonate with the lower centers of the body and the denser tissues. High pitched sounds resonate with the higher, less dense centers. Similarly, a guitar string will begin to vibrate when a companion string of the same pitch is plucked.

Another dimension to the sound of "Hum" is found in esoteric Tibetan Buddhism, in which spiritual teachings are

[27] Beaulieu, John. *Music and Sound in the Healing Arts*. p. 123.

[28] Capra, Fritjof. *The Tao of Physics*. p. 269.

summarized in the sound "Om Mani Padme Hum," which reverberates in chanting and prayer throughout the region. Stone offers insightful comments about this famous mantra. (Stone, *Polarity Therapy Vol. 2.* Book 5, p. 9).

Each part has a meaning: "Om" refers to gathering the outward tendencies and directing them up the chakras toward the eye center. "Mani" is the jewel or philosopher's stone of transmutation, by which the ordinary has the potential of transcendence. "Padme" is the natural, graceful evolutionary process symbolized in the opening of the lotus flower. "Hum" is transcending material illusion, above and beyond the eye center. As we hum, we momentarily partake in a profound and ancient system of spirituality whose cosmology is a source for Stone's Polarity Therapy.

Method

Find a comfortable posture in which to hum. The squat is excellent, especially the "wise man of old" posture, or another position in which you can comfortably place the thumbs or little fingers in the ears with the arms supported. Humming is done with the throat, mouth and jaw areas relaxed. The lips are barely closed and the teeth slightly parted.

Experiment with different pitches to intuitively choose the right one for the moment. Do that one pitch for one full breath or more, to completely experience that pitch. Then repeat, or do another, different pitch, higher or lower.

It is generally easier at first to feel the effects of different pitches in the face and skull. With time and practice, cultivating increased sensitivity, the effect can be felt in the torso as well.

Variations

In *Health Building* (p. 151-156), Stone describes humming to release the ear canal itself for people with ear problems and head noises. The little finger of each hand is placed in each ear and used to lift and dilate the canal. Pressing in different

Humming

This position can also be used for palpating your own cranial movement. Have your fingers touch the head so lightly that the hair is barely felt. The skull moves in slow, subtle cycles of expansion and contraction.

sides of the canal (front, back, up, down) gives different effects.

Hum different pitches until you feel the vibration in the selected area. Hum that pitch for a minute or so. When the focus is in the middle ear, press with both fingers equally. When the focus is more to one side, such as having symptoms on only one side, using one hand only may be preferred.

Humming is popular in an exercise classroom setting, as a great sound of varying pitches wells up in the group. It takes on increased impact with this increased volume and diversity.

Benefits
• Release and relaxation: the humming sound is both energizing and soothing, relaxing the nervous system and energizing the areas of the body which resonate with the sound's particular pitch.

• Humming pulls the attention inward; the effect is almost immediate. It is a great way to induce a centered feeling and to help shift from mental activity to a state of inner calm.

References
Stone, R. *Health Building*, pp. 150-151.
Stone, R. *Polarity Therapy Vol. 1*, Book 2. p. 79.

64. Ha!

A "Ha" sound contrasts greatly with humming. Rather than soothing, it has a stimulating and warming effect. Its forcefulness expels old gases from the lungs and creates the space for new, fresh air to come in. The diaphragm muscle moves powerfully and opens and balances itself. The expansive sound brings us into expression and movement with openness. Whereas "Om" and "Hum" are evolutionary, inward and stilling, "Ha" is involutionary, outward and creative. A loud, expressive sound like Ha can be quite liberating emotionally. The making of loud sounds, such as the cheering experienced at sporting events, can be very beneficial. Some teachers have suggested making loud Ha (or other) sounds when dealing with traffic, to release tension.

Method
See "Ha Breath" (page 70).

Variations
This sound can be quite loud and may not be appropriate in all situations. It is possible to do it with minimal sound, with only the "h-h-h" is audible.

Benefits
• Increases warmth and heat in the body.
• Stimulates self expression.
• Releases anger, facilitating expression of warmth and love.

65. Roar

The roar is a sustained sound that has many of the same benefits as the "Ha." It is warming, activating and releasing for the diaphragm, and encourages expression. The difference between this and the "Ha" is the steady sustained release of the sound: where the explosive "Ha" creates expression, the steady roar gives the power to sustain it.

Method

See Lion Roar (page 71).

66. Ah

A relaxed, sighing "Ah" is used to release breath and tension, assisting the eliminative, letting go process.

Method

Allow a deep full "a-a-h-h-h" to come out on your exhalation until the lungs are totally empty. As you get to the end of the breath, "blow out the candle" to completely expel the old air. Use the vibration of the sound to release tension and relax.

Benefits
- Assists complete exhalation. This is important in several exercises, such as the Cliffhanger (page 40) and some breathing exercises.
- Turns on the gestalt or reflex brain hemisphere so we can relax and not "try" so hard.
- Uses sound vibration to aid tension release in many exercises.

67. Laughter

Several authors, most notably Norman Cousins, have described the health benefits of laughter.

> Salivar immunoglobin A, which is believed to have a protective capacity against some viruses, increased significantly in the saliva of students who viewed a humorous videotape.[29]

---

[29] Cousins, Norman. *Head First*. p. 139. In *Anatomy of an Illness*, Cousins reported that 10 minutes of solid belly laughter gave him two hours of pain-free sleep during a severe illness. (p. 126).

In addition to dispelling tension, laughter has also been identified with thymus gland stimulation, reflexology benefits (with specific reflex points in the upper cheek area), relaxation of the brachial plexus and diaphragm, and other positive effects.

One simple game to make everyone in a group laugh is "Ha Ha." Lie on the floor, each person's head on the next person's stomach in a long chain. The first person loudly says "Ha," the next, "Ha Ha," and so on, each adding one more "Ha." It usually does not take long until it dissolves into laughter for all.

Brain Balancing

Just as the body has polarized currents and functions, so does the brain. The enormous subtlety and power of energy balancing for the brain is a relatively new area, and not found to great extent in Stone's writing. His system anticipates and complements the remarkable recent advances in the field.

Research into the brain's polarized functional relationships is entirely consistent with Stone's basic premises, and unveils large new areas for therapeutic application. The three principles seem to be perfectly reflected in the three dimensions: left/right being the Neutral Principle, top/bottom being the Yin Principle, and front/back being the Yang Principle. Applications of these correlations are discussed in a separate essay in Part Four.

People have a dominant side of brain function and sense function. For the eyes, a simple test to show which eye is habitually on is to make a small circle with both hands at arm's length, and sight through the circle to a distant object. Then close one eye at a time. With one eye closed, the image will be the same; with the other eye closed, it will move. Of course, nothing is moving; rather, one eye is dominant. The dominant eye is the one for which the image remains the same.

One side of the brain is more logical, sequential and language oriented. Edu-K calls this the "try" brain. This is usually, but not always, the left hemisphere. The other hemisphere is intuitive and holistic. In Edu-K this is called the "reflex" brain; this is usually, but not always the right hemisphere. A person who is not integrated in brain function, can have difficulty making full use of both sides.

Stone used the phrase "effortless effort" or "Wu Wei" to describe an integrated state, combining the effort of the try brain and the effortlessness of the reflex brain for optimum function.

Use of the term "switched on," suggesting an electrical switch, is appropriate, for when the brain is integrated, performance is dramatically improved: the image of a light bulb going on is based on proven theory here. This has been demonstrated in the use of brain integration techniques to teach drawing: students routinely break through to sudden major improvements when using these techniques.

The light bulb in the brain image, popularized in cartoons, is also supported by modern brain research. The front brain Conscious Associational Thinking (CAT) area is the site of new experience and insight, and has the seldom-used capacity to override habitual patterns.

> ...when artificially stimulated in test situations CAT registers a single specific response, LIGHT.[30]

Not surprisingly, it has been found that trauma and past experience play a key role in whether we are "switched on" or "switched off' in certain situations.

> In almost every instance, learning disabilities — popularly termed "dyslexia" — result from emotional stress at the time of learning, a stress so intense that the individual programs in a blind spot to a given learning skill due to fear, fear of pain, or pain itself.[31]

Energy balancing for the body is inevitably balancing for the brain as well, and vice versa. These exercises are subtle, powerful ways to work directly with activating smooth use of the whole brain, and enhancing the natural ability to switch back and forth into different functions as needed.

---

[30] Stokes and Whiteside. *One Brain.* Chapter 1, p. 22.

[31] *Ibid*, p. 3.

68. Re-Setting the Amygdalae

The amygdalae are two brain areas of critical importance in the stress response. Located on each side, one inch
beneath the temples and one inch behind the eye socket, at
the anterior end of the hippocampus, these almond-sized
brain centers constantly sort our experience to identify potential threats. The amygdalae pair is our early warning system
for general safety. In addition, the amygdalae are key players
in hormone balance, autonomic responses and other baseline
functions.

If any sensory input (sight, sound, smell, taste, touch or
extra-sensory perception) is identified by the amygdalae as
being potentially dangerous, an instant involuntary neuro-
chemical alarm system goes off and we begin a fight or flight
sequence before we have time to even identify the stressor.
The amygdalae record experiences throughout our lives and
use those experiences to compare present-time sensory perceptions. If we had particular threatening experiences as a
child, the amygdalae will sound the alarm if anything similar
happens later in life, just in case the current threat is real. For
example, if we had an upsetting event that approached from
the left at a particular time with particular sounds and colors,
later in life we are likely to become hyper-vigilant for events
from the left with similar characteristics.

A false alarm from the amygdalae can keep us in a fearful mode, with enormous negative consequences for our quality of life. People can be pre-programmed for stress responses
even if the danger is not actually real in the present. It would
be great to have a fresh start and be able to evaluate experiences on current value, instead of constantly reacting based
on long-ago threats.

For this reason, re-setting the amygdala offers the prom-
ise of liberation from the past, enabling us to be more realistic
and less prone to false alarms. Hypothetically the effect could

extend to ancestral or epigenetic factors, in addition to events that happened in our recent past.

Paul Lezchek (1920-1993) researched the subject in the 1950s and tested this method with many anxiety and depression patients, reporting great success. As a side note, Lezchek also removed his patients from electrical fields during the therapy, having them live off the grid in pure natural settings for a time to recover from their habitual stress states. He observed excellent, lasting results. Neil Slade and others have carried Lezchek's work into the present.

The method has some similarities to repetitive mindfulness practices for relief from anxiety and depression, but it is more focused on specific anatomy.

Method

Sitting comfortably, visualize the location, size, tone and presence of the amygdalae within your own head, to develop a felt-sense experience of this brain area. It can be palpated "by land" or "by sea," meaning using the soft tissue landmarks of the brain (anterior to the hippocampus in the tem-

Re-setting the Amygdala

Through visualization, the amygdalae can be oriented to the front (more modern) or back (more primitive).

poral lobe on each side) or the cerebrospinal fluid-filled temporal horns of the lateral ventricles. Take some time to try different approaches, to find out which method works for you. With practice, you can learn to visualize your amygdalae accurately and quickly.

Note any perceived differences between left and right amygdalae; one may seem more forward/rearward, elevated/descended, smaller/larger, more active/passive, or any other comparative characteristic. In particular, notice whether the amygdalae seem more oriented to the front or back. According to Slade, the front (behind the forehead) represents a higher order of response, engaging the more sophisticated prefrontal cortex, whereas a rear orientation (inside the lower occiput) represents a more primitive response, engaging the instinctual, "law of the jungle" centers in the brainstem.

Once you have a sense of the amygdalae, use your imagination to picture nudging them forward. Imagine that the inner surface of the forehead is a movie screen with a captivating story being displayed, and the amygdalae are people in the audience leaning forward in fascination. Similarly, imagine that a soft feather is placed behind the amygdalae, tickling them to shift more anteriorly in the head.

This practice may seem odd at first, but gradually we can increase our capacity for perception of the amygdalae's location and condition.

Repetition is the key, to give the brain a chance to develop for this purpose, so at least a daily ten-minute practice for at least two weeks is needed to start to get the benefit. At first we may not be able to sense an inner brain area, but after two weeks the location will probably become more obvious and the difference between forward and rearward orientation will become increasingly clear.

Benefits
- Lowers the tendency to involuntarily over-react fearfully to life situations.

• Gradually cultivates equanimity and capacity for being in the present instead of the past and future.

References
Slade, Neil. *The Frontal Lobes Supercharge*.
Slade, Neil. *Brain Magic*. pp. 12 ff

Related Exercises
Brain Buttons (p. 140)

69. Lazy Eights For Eyes

In Lazy Eights for Eyes we activate both sides of the brain, both eyes, and the natural link between brain, eye and hand coordination. This exercise makes use of the concept of "crossing the midline." For the eyes, crossing the midline refers to the process by which we switch primary use from one brain hemisphere to the other as the eyes move across a visual field. For many people, crossing the midline is difficult, and activities such as reading and coordination suffer.

Method

This fun activity can be done several different ways. The simplest way requires no extra materials and can be done

Lazy Eights for Eyes

Use a large version of this shape to trace the Lazy Eights. Use a figure at least two feet wide, traced at full arm's length distance. Either follow your thumb or use crayons of markers to draw the Lazy Eight. Go up in the middle and down on the sides.

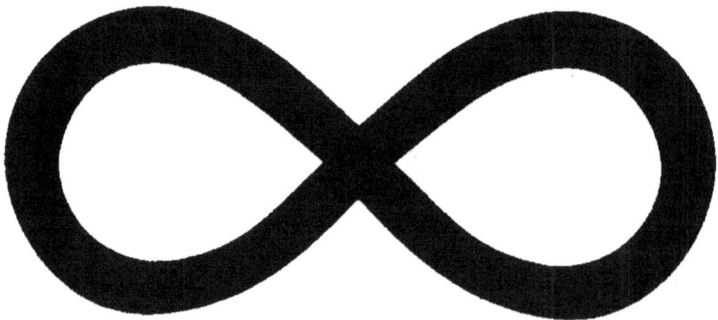

anywhere. Stand or sit comfortably. Hold one hand extended in front of the nose, thumb up on the midline in the center of the body. Fix your sight on the thumbnail. Now move the thumb in a lazy eight (∞) shape, by moving it up the midline and circling to the left. Make a full circle back to center and then another circle over to the right.

Continue this lazy eight motion and follow each part of the movement with your eyes. The head remains centered and relaxed and the eyes follow slowly so they move easily and do not miss any section of the eight.

After eight times or more, use the other hand to draw the lazy eight, again following continuously with the eyes, head remaining centered. After eight times or more, draw the lazy eight with both hands together.

This can also be done with colored pencils, markers or crayons on a big sheet of paper or chalkboard. Make sure to keep the nose as the midline and follow with your eyes. Another possibility is using a child's toy car or train that has a figure eight track.

Variation: The Elephant

Crossing the midline can be a problem in hearing as well. For this situation, the Dennisons developed "the Elephant" in which the head rests on the shoulder and moves as the whole arm traces lazy eights.

Benefits
- Eases reading. This exercise has given dramatic benefit to people with reading problems.
- Improved hand/eye coordination.
- Connects and balances left and right brain functions.
- Gives a sense of stability and calm.

References
Dennison, Paul and Gail. *Brain Gym*, p. 5.
Stokes, Gordon and Whiteside, Daniel. *One Brain*, Chapter 8, pp. 16 ff.

70. Dennison Laterality Repatterning

Repatterning is a term for the brain integration therapies created by Paul and Gail Dennison. In Repatterning, simple movements are employed to activate both sides of the brain and improve communication between them.

Repatterning is often used in relation to a particular task. Often we want to be good at something, but find it just gets more difficult the more we try to do it. Similarly, we may know our attitude is defeating us in a particular task, yet we are unable to change to an attitude that would be successful.

In this situation it is sometimes said, "You don't really want to change or you would do it." To the observer, this seems the only plausible reason for failure. But the problem is not so simple. The unfortunate person can be locked in a "homolateral" (single-sided or same-sided) state, with inter-communication of the two brain hemispheres shut down or short-circuited. The more this person tries, the more difficult it actually does get. The try hemisphere (usually, but not always the left) is working hard detailing and organizing, but the reflex hemisphere (usually, but not always the right) is shut off from the action.

A person may be homolateral for certain situations or actions and not others, often in response to childhood trauma and experience. One might be well integrated as a skier and homolateral as a cook, or good at writing, but poor at sports. Lost skills can be re-integrated with this process.

Usually this method is taught using a biofeedback system called muscle checking. For more information on this, see the Bibliography in the back of the book. References here to Kinesiology are the beginning of a very large subject, and further study of details is highly recommended to the Polarity student.

In this exercise, the reflex brain hemisphere is connected with a movement that uses both sides of the body at once. We then activate the try brain hemisphere, which is connected with a movement using one side only. Then the two parts are integrated for whole brain functioning.

The movement consists of marching in place in two particular ways, and then bringing the hands together. Bringing the hands together prompts the two brain hemispheres to begin communication. The actual link is found in the central brain in the commissures, particularly the largest, the corpus callosum. The hand movement represents the movement of messages back and forth across this bridge. In Polarity terms, the connection of right and left in the neutral pole (the hands) completes a circuit, inducing a similar connection in the positive pole (the brain).

In addition to movement, sound and sight are employed. For sound, the reflex (usually right) brain is activated by humming, while the try (usually left) brain is activated by counting. Many people can actually feel the difference, and can readily identify which side is active in each activity. When humming, hum on only one note. When counting, count crisply and clearly without singsong or rhythm.

The reflex brain is activated by looking up and the try brain is activated by looking down.

Method

If you are repatterning for a specific action, think of it or do it and notice how your body feels. Now begin marching in place with opposite arm and leg moving simultaneously, called the "cross crawl." Notice how that feels. Then do the homolateral crawl (same arm and leg) and notice how that feels. Often the cross crawl will feel more awkward when we are switched off. It requires using both brain hemispheres at once and becomes difficult when there is a lack of integration.

Now begin the actual re-patterning movements by humming, looking up and cross crawling in place. The cross crawl replicates a stage of crawling for young children, which is critical to brain development. As you look up, look to the

Dennison Laterality Repatterning

First Phase
"Cross Crawl"
Hum and Look Up

Second Phase
"Homolateral Crawl"
Count and Look Down

left, the center and the right, moving only the eyes. Find the direction that makes marching easiest. Continue looking in that direction, humming, and marching until you feel easy and natural with the movement. This becomes your easy way or high gear.

Next, look down while counting and doing a puppet march, in which the same side arm and leg rise together. This is called the "homolateral crawl." Look down in the direction opposite that which was easy during cross crawling. Homolateral crawl until it becomes awkward or tiring. This becomes your low gear.

Integration Metaphor

After both marching in place movements, including appropriate eye placement and sound, do the Integration Metaphor. Stretch the arms out wide in front and slowly bring the hands together until they are clasping. Hold this position until you feel complete. Clasping the hands symbolizes renewed and enhanced communication between left and right sides of the brain.

Now reach your arms out to the sides with hands open. Imagine one brain hemisphere in each hand, getting ready to come together. Slowly move the hands together until clasping, fingers interlocked, holding until you feel complete. Take your time and move however feels right for you.

A therapist can monitor the craniosacral rhythm as the hands are being held. The person may be in a craniosacral stillpoint, processing for some time. Many people can feel the energy releases happening as tingles, pulses or brain activity and it is clear to them when they are complete.

Finally, cross crawl and look in all directions, then do the homolateral crawl while looking in all directions. Then briefly cross crawl again. Always finish with the cross crawl.

Last, do some version of the original activity, and repeat the two methods of marching. Notice the difference from the beginning, to establish or anchor the change.

Variations

For a quick integration you can first hum, then count, and familiar tune (such as "Row your Boat" or "Happy Birthday"). Make sure to look different directions: up, down, right, left, center. Experiment with eyes open and eyes closed. This is fun and can be effective for easing a difficult activity. Also, in a classroom situation, it helps people feel the hidden machinery at work in consciousness.

Benefits
- Improves ability to function with effortless effort or ease of action, especially for attitudes or activities which are chronically difficult.
- Release from feelings of blockage and obstruction.

References
Dennison, Paul and Gail. *Edu-K for Kids*, p. 20.
Dennison, Paul and Gail. *Brain Gym*, p. 4.

71. Mudras for Three Principles and Five Elements

Mudras are positions and gestures of the body and hands that have energetic meaning and function. Mudras have a long history in Asian cultures, being used in meditation, Hatha Yoga, ritual ceremonies and dance, and other applications.

Mudras can often be seen in depictions of Buddha, Quan Yin and other saints and mythological characters in Eastern spiritual traditions. Buddha is often shown with right hand (Yang) raised and projecting out while the left hand (Yin) is palm upward and receptively held on the lap.

In *The Last Supper*, Leonardo da Vinci showed Jesus using this left-hand-up, right-hand-down positioning. Completing the symbolic tableaux, all the apostles on the left of the painting have matching downturned palms, and all the figures on the right have matching upraised palms.

Try these hand positions to create a sense of wellbeing. Each one has particular effects, so experiment with each one in different situations to find out what works best for you.

Three Principles
This hand position is used to balance the Three Principles, especially during quiet relaxation or meditation. The left

hand represents Yin and right hand represents Yang. The right thumb (Yang/Ether) is contained and protected by the left fist, and the rest of the right hand surrounds and protects the left hand. This position promotes stability, equanimity and interdependence of the body's dual-pole energy system. It can be used to re-set the system in both worldly and spiritual contexts, such as when waiting for an appointment or during a calming practice.

Three Principles
Left hand encloses the right thumb

Five Elements

Gently connecting all five fingertips of one hand to their corresponding fingertips on the other hand completes the circuit for each element. This enhances the flow and drains surplus charge while also augmenting deficient charge in any element.

A similar concept is used in Polarity Therapy bodywork, most often with the practitioners touching their clients' toes with their own corre-

Five Elements
Fingertips complete the elemental circuits

sponding fingertips. The concept is discussed in several places in Stone's writing. Similar to the Three Principles mudra, holding this pose helps re-set the energy field. It should be held long enough for a pulsation to be detected in each fingertip, indicating that the circuit has more flow. Normally this takes at least two or three minutes.

Polarity Circle

Holding hands in a circle is often done by groups to create a sense of communal inclusion and coherence. Examples include joining hands in prayer at the dinner table or standing together in a closing circle after an event.

To heighten the effect using Polarity Therapy or Taoist principles, have the people put their right palms facing down and their left palms facing up, representing the dual action of Yang and Yin, respectively. For fun, have a group just hold hands in a circle randomly, then after the effect can be perceived, change to the Three Principles approach and wait, to determine if a difference in coherence can be detected.

Polarity Circle
Right palm down,
left palm up

Benefits (for all Polarity mudras)
• Soothing and centering; good for recovery from over-stimulating events
• Good position for meditation or waiting.

References
Stone, R. *Polarity Therapy Vol. 1*, Book 3, p. 24.

Sha, Zhi Gang. *Tao Song and Tao Dance: Sacred Sound, Movement and Power from the Source for Longevity and Transformation of All Life.* pp. 15 & 17. The Taoist versions of these two poses are slightly different.

Related Exercises
Sensory Balance (p. 122)
Cook's Hookups (p. 127)

Breathing that Balances

We have never seen a disturbed person who did not
have some abnormality of breathing.[32]

Breathing is an essential part of energy exercise. Awareness and development of breath is an age-old component of
all energy-based healing systems. Well known in yogic and
martial arts practices, it is present in every tradition. We believe full and balanced breathing is a benefit for all health
conditions and often the first and greatest self-help step any
person can take.

> While working with the S.A.G.E. project, I and oth-
> ers experimented with a variety of growth tech-
> niques and practices in an attempt to revitalize the
> minds and bodies of older men and women. Among
> the practices that we experimented with were relax-
> ation training, electromyograph bio-feedback, deep
> breathing, Hatha yoga, bodymind awareness exer-
> cises, massage, Feldenkrais exercises, individual
> counseling, meditation, T'ai Chi, music therapy, and
> Gestalt Therapy. After the first year of practice and
> research, we interviewed the participants about
> which of the techniques seemed to be most effective
> for them in the restoration of emotional energy,
> physical well-being, and feelings of interpersonal
> connectedness.[33]

The concept of Prana is an important part of breathing
for energy benefit. Prana (the East Asian equivalent is Ch'i or
Qi) is a word for the subtle cosmic life force which rides on
air, sunlight and moving water. Just as the cells need oxygen,
the energy systems need Prana. It is thought to be absorbed

---

[32] Kurtz & Prestera, *The Body Reveals*, p. 83.

[33] Dychtwald, Ken. *Bodymind.* p. 147.

through a membrane at the top of the nasal passage, hence the emphasis on inhalation through the nose. Some yogis are reputed to live on breath alone, obtaining life energy from Prana only.

Therapeutic breathing can be differentiated into its three parts: inhalation, exhalation and rest. This cycle mirrors the three stages of energy movement, or three principles. Many people breathe unevenly, over- or under- emphasizing one or another part. Thus they are habitually over-expanded or under-filled or without stillness. These characteristics of breathing can be read as an accurate way of self-discovery, indicating imbalance in the system. Breath indicates inner conditions on mental, emotional and physical levels.

On the popular health issue front, many disruptive flora (such as the fungus *Candida Albicans*) are anaerobic, thriving without oxygen. As we oxygenate the body through deep inhalation, these make way for healthier flora. Oxygen is also needed for the chemical reaction required to burn fat or use energy properly. For weight loss, this is accomplished by aerobic exercise: deep and full breathing supports such a program.

Exhalation is equally important, if more subtle. It is the essential elimination of cellular waste. Exhalation is associated with the critical emotional function of letting go, an eventual goal (after first facing the pain) in the recovery from emotional trauma. More people seem to have trouble with exhalation than inhalation, perhaps due to the materialistic nature of modern times: we live in a time in which Yang qualities are glorified, and Yin is poorly understood and under-appreciated.

After the exhale is a moment of rest. In our accelerated lives, this rest point is sometimes forgotten. This indicates a loss of neutrality and stillness emotionally, characteristic in a person caught up in busy activities with no time to contemplate new or deeper meanings. This is also found in people with childhood trauma of such severity as to create disassociation of the mind, emotions, and body from each other. Locked in to habitual patterns of reaction to the trauma, it is difficult to rest or be neutral.

Energy exercises offer a general opportunity to become more aware of breathing, and to practice full, balanced breathing using the whole body. In addition, several specific breathing exercises are offered here.

72. Inhale 2, Hold 8, Exhale 4

This is a stimulating, oxygenating breath. Take the time for a breathing break. Sit, lie or stand in a comfortable posture in a place where the air is the freshest available. Inhale strongly and deeply to a slow count of 2. Hold for a count of 8. Exhale fully for a count of 4. Repeat five to ten times. Slow exhalation is relaxing, strong exhalation is stimulating.

Reference
Robbins, *Unlimited Power*, p. 171.

73. Belly Breathing

This is a relaxing and soothing breath. Rest the hands on the abdomen. Inhale slowly and deeply, feeling the belly fill up like a balloon. As you exhale, purse your lips slightly and breathe out in short little puffs as if you are keeping a feather in the air. Feel the rhythm of the belly softly rising and falling. To take the air deeper, arch your back after inhaling.

References
Dennison, Paul and Gail. *Brain Gym*, p. 12.
Barhydt, Harrison and Elizabeth. *Self-Help for Stress and Pain*, p. 43.
Lowen, Alexander. *The Way to Vibrant Health*, p. 99.

74. Watch Your Breath

This technique brings relaxation through contemplation. Find a comfortable position and close the eyes. Concentrate on the breath, without any intention of changing it in any way. Watch what it does. It will adjust without conscious effort.

75. Alternate Nostril Breathing

This yogic breathing exercise facilitates balance of the right and the left nostrils, brain hemispheres and sympathetic and parasympathetic nervous systems. During the day we normally switch breathing for time periods (when healthy, every 50 minutes to 2 hours), so that one nostril and then the other predominates. The right (Yang side) nostril is activating in its effect and the left (Yin side) nostril is relaxing.

Breathe and watch the breath. Determine which nostril you are currently using. Next, purposefully alternate nostrils by using the thumb and forefinger to close off one nostril and then the other by pressing just above the flared portion of the nostril. Close off the right nostril with the thumb. Inhale and then exhale through the left nostril. Switch so the forefinger is closing off the left nostril. Inhale and exhale through the right nostril. Continue this process and notice the effects.

This exercise can take some time to perfect. While it sounds simple, it is subtle and profound. Do it daily for a week, to develop sensitivity and skill.

Benefits
- Re-establishes balanced breathing.
- Concentrates attention.

Reference
Stone, R. *The Mystic Bible*, p. 114.

Exercises and Practices for Elimination

Inevitably, exercise programs and elimination programs overlap. In our progress toward better energy and vitality, increased function of the elimination systems is very significant. There are five systems of elimination, one for each of the five elements or chakras: Earth/bowels, Water/urine and lymph, Fire/sweat, Air/carbon dioxide exhalation, and Ether/expression of feelings. Lack of function of any of these will eventually be fatal, and declining health is accompanied by difficulty in any of these elimination pathways. Exercise can play a part in all of these areas, with Fire and Air the most obvious, as any physical activity will increase perspiration and breathing rate.

Elimination pathways for each Element	
Earth	Bowels
Water	Urine
Fire	Sweat
Air	CO_2
Ether	Expression

Diet

A brief statement on diet is appropriate here. There are two approaches to take when improving elimination functions: enhancing removal, and reducing the toxicity of material taken in. Both are important. For the second approach, we advocate a lacto-vegetarian or vegan diet, in keeping with Stone's teaching:

> The proteins of flesh meats and eggs have many by-products in them, such as... wastes of the animal system. These must be eliminated in order to maintain health. (Stone, *Polarity Therapy Vol. 1.* Appendix, p. 115)

"LiverFlush" Recipe	**"Polarity Tea" Recipe**
One Serving: Combine in a blender: 6 oz. Orange Juice (apple may be substituted), 1 TB cold-pressed olive oil, 1 TB fresh lemon juice, 1 inch chopped fresh ginger, 1 or 2 peeled cloves garlic, cayenne to taste. For low sugar version, use water instead of juice. Experiment with proportions!	Two Servings: Mix together seeds and roots, equal parts licorice root, fennel seed, fenugreek seed and double parts flax seed. Bring 2+ cups water to a boil, add 1 heaping TB of this mixture and let boil/steep for five minutes. For convenience, make a larger amount and store refrigerated. Then add 1/2 TB dried peppermint leaves and cover, steep for five more minutes.

There are many good reasons to be a vegetarian: our favorite books on the subject are Robbins' *Diet for a New America* and McDougall's *The McDougall Plan*.

Stone taught extensively on using the vegetarian diet for specific purposes. He described two sub-categories of vegetarian eating, the "Health Building" and "Purifying" Diets. For elimination and cleansing, the Purifying diet, consisting of raw and cooked vegetables or fruit (minimizing protein, starch, and oil and avoiding salt and sugar altogether) has been proven to be effective. Stone also recommended an orange juice/olive oil "Liverflush" followed by an herbal tea formula which has since been called Polarity Tea, to complete the cleansing program.

Deep Bodywork

There is a direct link between deep pressure on the body and elimination. This was discussed earlier in the context of "Touches that Balance." Each Principle has a corresponding touch: light and balancing for Neutral, vigorous and stimulating for Yang, deep and changing for Yin. Elimination is a primary function of the Yin Principle, and deep touch amplifies and stimulates this, the Yin part of the energy system promoting elimination on all levels.

76. The Box

Stone used the Box as a way to put deep pressure on the feet. As we discussed in "Touches that Balance" in noting the predominance of Yin therapy, energy tends to slow down as it gets more distant from the core. Energy is able to go out, but less able to get back. The pelvis and the feet, as the negative poles of the torso and the whole body, respectively, are the locations of this tendency to become fixed. In using the box, we forcibly soften this dense and congested field, while also engaging the shoulders (via the muscular activity of the hand support) and torso (by moving in various positions). Since all parts of the body have reflexes in the feet, the Box can be used to facilitate elimination and change in any of the five elemental zones.

To create a box, an edge and a hand support are needed. The edge should have a slightly rounded corner, without danger of splinters, about 4 to 8 inches above the floor. This

The Box
This shows a simple way to create a Box
at home, with a 4x4 post and a doorway.

can be a framed box of wood, the edge of a stair or a large timber. The hand support can be a bar fastened to the wall, a staircase bannister, a door handle or the edges of a door frame with a stout broom handle wider than the doorway, or any other invention for the purpose.

Method

To use the box, step on the edge and experiment with different postures: leaning back, squatting and shifting from side to side. Breathe deeply and make sound.

This can be painful, and each individual has to set his or her own pace. You can start with thick socks and work up to bare feet. If the feet are found to be very rigid and sore, do the Box or something like it daily.

Benefits

- Deep pressure is applied on the feet, while colon reflexes in wrists, calves and neck are simultaneously activated.
- Use the Box when you want changes to occur, on any level.

References

Stone, R. *Health Building*, p. 167.
Lowen, Alexander. *The Way to Vibrant Health*, p. 76.

Earth Elimination Exercises

Exercise is only part of the methods available for improving elimination for the Earth Element. Herbal programs, the use of psyllium as a bulking agent, the drinking of adequate amounts of water, avoiding animal foods and cultivating an attitude of relaxation and letting go are all worthy of mention. Robert Gray's *Colon Health Handbook* is highly recommended.

77. Squatting

The Squat is a key defense against colon problems, not only for its already described value as an exercise. The topic of posture during defecation has been discussed by many authors, who invariably struggle against the indelicacy of the subject and people's reluctance to discuss, much less change, such intimate personal habits. The modern toilet has been identified with a host of modern health problems, such as a malfunctioning ileocecal valve (one study estimated this at 80% of the population),[34] constricted colon (constipation), autointoxication, prolapsis of organs, swelling of the abdomen, and several degenerative diseases, including cancer.

This is not a new debate: a line of brave doctors has preached the same message throughout the century, to no avail. In the 1980s, Dr. Welles of San Diego took up the campaign, including designing and selling devices to facilitate squatting during defecation and in exercise.

An agile person can squat on an existing conventional toilet, while others can design or acquire appropriate fixtures (platform, hand rails, etc.) for their most frequently used facilities. If squatting is impossible, one can lift up one or both feet to the seat while still seated. If one foot is used, the left (descending colon side) is recommended, to support the abdominal wall. An easier alternative is to have a stool next to the toilet to hold the foot somewhat raised.

78. Skin Brushing

> Five minutes per day of skin brushing is easily worth 30 minutes of vigorous physical exercise in this respect [colon therapy].[35]

The interrelationship of skin, colon and the lymphatic system is a complex subject, whether considered in terms of conventional anatomy or energy theory.

Skin brushing, if done regularly, is a profoundly beneficial exercise. It activates the colon, assists in the discharge of old fecal matter, accelerates the flow and elimination of lymphatic fluid and imparts a lustrous tone to the entire body.

[34] Welles, *The Hidden Crime of the Porcelain Throne.* p. 1.
[35] Gray, Robert. *The Colon Health Handbook.* p. 23.

At home, use a long-handled (so the back can be reached) natural hair brush to stroke the bare skin evenly for about 3 to 5 minutes each day. The skin and brush should be dry, and a systematic, one directional movement should be used. Go from the extremities toward the abdomen. Brush up the legs, then up the arms, then down the torso, etc. Sweep all surfaces except the face. The pressure used is very light, and the exercise is not to be confused with skin scrubbing or exfoliation.

79. Colon Reflexes

There are several reflexology opportunities to stimulate the colon. The colon has overlapping relationships, primarily the Neutral Principle (Chest-Colon-Calves) and Earth Element (Neck-Bowels-Knees). The most frequently cited colon reflexes in Polarity Therapy are the muscles of the calves, and the feet (in the center area on the bottom, and between the fourth and fifth toes on the top and bottom).

Using the fists to exercise the calf muscle is described on page 65. In addition, calf lengthening (page 201) has a toning colon effect. Squatting is especially beneficial for the colon, bringing chest-colon-calves (the three poles of the Neutral Principle) into closest possible proximity for efficient energy movement and amplification.

For the feet, gentle or deep rubbing has a stimulating effect. Press along the web of the foot between the toes, holding on sore spots. For the bottom of the foot, more pressure can be created by standing on the edge of a board (see The Box, page 191), book, bottle, can or other object (a wooden "footsie roller" is made commercially for the purpose).

Another way to press the feet is to sit in a kneeling position, with buttocks back near the heels. Use the knuckles to press in on the calves, then continue down into the foot. The colon reflex area follows the main arch, just below the ball of the foot. Start on the right foot and press up to the outside arch area, then across the foot to the arch instep. Continue on the left foot from instep to outside of foot and down. This path mirrors the ascending, transverse and descending path of the colon.

Stone also mentions stimulation of the tongue as a colon reflex. Like the ear, the tongue is a complex combination of reflexes for the whole torso. This stimulation can be done by pressing the tongue firmly in all directions, by creating suction, by scraping with the teeth (especially the sides of the tongue) or a device made for the purpose, by contact with a tongue depressor and other means.

Benefits
- Stimulates colon.
- General revitalization for the whole body: colon function has a central significance in all systems. Some authors (Gray, Jensen) have said colon distress is a factor in all degenerative disease.

References
Stone, R. *Polarity Therapy Vol. 1*, Book 1, pp. 48-49, Book 2, pp. 17, 81-82.
Stone, R. *Polarity Therapy Vol. 2*, pp. 150-151, 183-184, 199, 20l.

80. Valve Tapping

A rhythmic tapping with the fingertips at the corners of the colon is effective for general relaxation and for stimulating peristalsis and colon valve function. This technique was shown to one of our editors by an Ayurvedic doctor in India.

Method
Tap with light or medium pressure over the ileocecal valve on the right and over the sigmoid valve on the left. These are located on either side of the front abdomen, two inches below and to either side of the navel. Take your time and breathe deeply during the tapping. Afterwards, relax and hold the spot lightly with one hand, while touching the other side with the other hand as a balance.

Related Exercises
Self Organ Drain, p. 70.

Massage the colon with small circular contacts, from right to left following the colon. This direct contact should not be used if there is pain or degenerative disease in the abdomen.

Water Elimination Exercises

The water system responds to healthful liquids, and to movement. Many people are dehydrated, especially in the dry environments of forced air office buildings. Water, herb tea and juices should always be kept nearby for refreshment, using up to two quarts of water each day for a cleansing program. Sugared, caffeinated or alcoholic beverages supply polluted water: the water is used, but unhealthy side effects are experienced.

Movement is the primary mechanical way that the lymphatic system takes waste materials away from the cells. The lymph also receives some pumping action from its duct system. Stone makes the larger point that circulation of fluids in the body originates in the deep energy currents, the pulsation of expansion and contraction. Mechanical actions, including the heart, lymphatic ducts, peristalsis and one-way valves, etc. are secondary reflections of pulsating energy, the subtle basis of all pumping action.

Water: Essential to Brain Balance

Being composed primarily of water, the body naturally needs water to maintain balance. This is especially important in brain function. The electrochemical process depends on correct water levels for proper function. Often the correction to feelings of sluggishness or confusion can be as simple as drinking some water. Avoiding dehydration is especially significant under stress, and in lifestyles in which frequent drinking is difficult. For example, a closed-air office building with a fast pace of activity will be especially conducive to dehydration.

---

81. Rebounding (Home Trampoline)

Of all possible movement options, rebounding stands out as the most beneficial for the lymphatic system. Rebounding is light or vigorous jumping on a small trampoline. Its efficiency is due to the up and down motion, in which a miniature weightlessness/gravity-force cycle is created. At the top of the jump, upward momentum balances downward gravity, and a split second of artificial weightlessness is achieved. At this moment, a minuscule de-pressurized expansion occurs throughout the body.

At the bottom of the cycle, momentum and gravity are combined against the resistance of the bouncing surface to create a slight "G-force" situation, causing minute pressurized contraction throughout the body. Thus rebounding facilitates the expansion and contraction of all systems, creating cellular breathing to assist drainage of waste from cells, and movement of liquids through lymphatic channels.

The energy exercise classroom will benefit by having a few rebounders, with one or two located by a secure rail for older people to hold while they bounce. Even the slightest movement is beneficial, improving vitality and circulation without excessive shock to the joints.

Fire Elimination

Sweat is the goal here, so active movement is the primary method. Other alternatives are steam rooms and saunas, and swimming or exercising in medium or warmer temperature water. We are partial to natural hot springs for this purpose. Saunas are more effective because more sweat is eliminated in the dry environment.

It has been found, incidentally, that exercising in water does not burn fat effectively and is a lower priority method of exercise if weight loss is a primary goal.

Air Elimination

This function is covered in the section on breathing, beginning on page 185. Emphasis is on the exhale, and on an attitude of letting go.

Ether Elimination

The Ether Center at the throat is the location of self-expression, discrimination, longing and grief. Managing these are all goals of many therapy systems. "Emotional constipation" of not being able to speak one's feelings, whether for internal or external reasons, is a serious prelude to health problems.

The Ether Element is challenged by modern conditions leading to alienation. Many people find themselves with no one to talk to authentically about deep life experiences. Chronic alienation affects the Ether Element profoundly.

Etheric elimination uses expression of feelings and other ways of making sound. The Lion Roar and Ha Breath are examples of supportive exercises that have been discussed.

Music

Music had its own section earlier. For purposes of elimination, music can assist in the evocation of feelings, provide a forum for expression (choral singing is especially enjoyable, and a part of holidays and religious events for good reasons from an energy perspective) and encourage liberating movement.

Certain kinds of movement can also be effective:

> Rhythmic expressions of song and dance, which use all the bodily forces and muscles for expression, free the emotions by naturally liberating the energy blocks, suppressions, frustrations and stagnations.
> (Stone, *Health Building.* p. 108)

Lengthening

These simple lengthening exercises are for specific muscle release. They make a good preparation for some of the more complex postures, and can be used with bodywork to accomplish with leverage that which would be hard to do with pressure. Re-read the introduction to lengthening at the beginning of the book. Remember never to strain or bounce into these postures. Hold, at the edge of release, and wait for the muscle to let go on its own and reset at a new length. It is very useful to know the location (including origin, insertion point, and tendons) of each specific muscle, and the desired direction of lengthening.

Most people have one or two particular muscles that are tighter than the others. You can figure out which muscles among the following are most important for you, and help create a habit of working on those one or two lengthening postures. If the worst case is improved, all the others (and the whole body) will benefit.

82. Inner Thigh Lengthening

The origin of the inner thigh muscle is in front of the pubic bone. The insertion is along the thigh, beginning just below the hip and going down to just below the knee on the inside of the lower leg.

Method

Start with the feet spread wider than shoulder width. Decide which leg will be straightened for lengthening. Keep the foot of this leg turned out to avoid straining the inner knee ligament. Place the hands on the thigh above the knee of the opposite leg. Shift the hips toward the bent leg and as you bend into that knee you will feel the inner thigh lengthening on the opposite straight leg. Go to a point of tension that feels like it will allow the muscles to release, let go and reset. Then,

Inner Thigh Lengthening

bend further for another level of release or come out of the posture. Take a moment to quietly experience the new lengthening.

83. Calf Lengthening I

The soleus is a part of the calf muscle, deeper and inside the gastrocnemius. The origin is just below the inner knee on the back of the leg and the insertion is at the heel.

Method

Stand with the feet in a medium-length stride, one foot forward and the other foot back, feet facing straight forward. Bend slowly into both knees and focus on the area of the origin and insertion of the soleus in the back leg. Feel the tension of the lengthening in the Achilles tendon. Stop at the edge of release and hold, waiting for the muscle to let go and reset. Repeat with a deeper bend for further lengthening or come to standing and experience the new length in the calf.

Calf Lengthening I: Soleus

84. Calf Lengthening II

The origin of the gastrocnemius muscle is on the back of the leg just above the knee, and the insertion is in the middle of the back of the heel. This is the large double bellied muscle of the calves which lifts the heel in walking. It is also the bottom of the tendon guard reflex, the body's instinctive response to stress. Wise runners lengthen here before starting.

Method

Place the feet in a long stride with one foot forward and one foot back. Place the hands on the thigh of the forward leg and lean over the front knee, keeping the back flat and maintaining balance as you go. Spread the feet as far as needed to keep a tension in the back calf that is on the edge of release. Wait for the muscles to let go to a new length. Then, lean even more or push the back heel further down for more release, or come to standing and do the opposite leg. When complete, come to standing and take a moment to experience the new feeling of length.

Calf Lengthening II: Gastrocnemius

85. Hamstring Lengthening

These muscles are located in the thigh. The origin is at the lowest part of the hip bone and the insertion is at the top of the lower leg just below the back of the knee.

This muscle is commonly tight due to the customs of sitting in chairs and rarely walking barefoot. It is also part of the tendon guard reflex, in which the back side of the body tightens in response to stress. In a high-stress lifestyle, this area can become permanently over-tightened. This position,

Hamstring Lengthening

which has similarities to and can be done with the Pyramid, is a beneficial daily routine first thing in the morning.

Method

Stand with the legs more than shoulder width apart. Place the hands on the thighs just above the knees. Keep the back flat as you lean forward. Push with the hands and keep lifting the buttocks toward the ceiling, this separates the origin and insertion points. Notice the tension being created in the back of the upper thighs. Go to the edge of release and wait for the muscles to let go and reset. Push more for further release. When done, come to standing and feel this new hamstring length. Notice how overall posture has been affected.

86. Psoas Lengthening

The psoas is a major structural muscle; its origin runs along the spine from the vertebra at the lowest ribs (12th thoracic vertebrae) through all the vertebrae of the curve of the lower back (lumbar vertebrae). The insertion is in the front, on the inside of the upper thigh bone on a level with the pubic bone. This is the muscle used to lift the leg in walking. This lengthening can be used to accompany five pointed star Polarity Therapy techniques.

Because this muscle goes from the front (of the thigh) to the back, tightness here forces a curve (Lordosis) in the lower back. This tips the pelvis to make the shortest possible distance from front to back. Lengthening the psoas can thus release the lower back and allow the pelvis to return to proper alignment.

Method

Stand with the feet in a stride position, one foot in front, one foot in back, both feet facing forward. Allow both knees to bend and the back heel to lift, thrusting the pelvis forward and keeping the back straight. Focus on the front inner thigh area. Feel the tension reaching into the psoas.

If you do not feel the tension in the front of the pelvis, spread the feet further apart. Make sure the pelvis is thrust forward by pulling the navel in toward the back and if necessary squeezing the buttocks. Contraction in back creates extension in front.

Psoas Lengthening

Hold at the edge of release until the muscle releases and resets. When done, stand up and feel this new openness.

Practices for Autonomic NS First Aid

87. Body-Low-Slow-Loop Practice (BLSL)

Anna Chitty had the original insight to create this practice, after her study of Somatic Experiencing. BLSL has become one of our most useful methods in both classes and private sessions. This and the subsequent practice are reprinted from *Dancing with Yin and Yang* (2013).

This practice provides Autonomic Nervous System (ANS) first aid in the simplest possible way. It helps clients get started in self-regulation, and introduces the body-centered approach to people who have not studied trauma resolution. BLSL is a simple exercise that anyone can learn and apply safely and effectively with minimal training. It is not a cure-all for solving autonomic distress or a substitute for more substantial therapy; instead it is a first-aid method that can be learned for general soothing, and then deployed in a time of high stress when other resources are not available.

Regularly performing BLSL daily for ten to fifteen minutes can help gradually overcome the residual effects of trauma without having to go into the details of what happened. This practice has been very effective for many people in restoring the ANS back to an approximation of its original design. It seems to take about six weeks of regular practice to get the full benefits.

Each word in the phrase Body-Low-Slow-Loop is one stage of the process:

Body

In this first step, we direct clients to bring their attention into the body and to notice their sensations. Bringing the attention into the body, instead of the thoughts or feelings that may be present, can be a revelation in itself. The mind becomes the audience, the body the performer. The sensations that initially attract attention could be caused simply by sensory nerves detecting contact with surfaces due to gravity, or

just the movement of breath.[36] We all have these basic sensations, all the time.

In addition to the ever-present normal sensations, the
initial primary (or loudest) sensations could also be after-ef-
fects of recent or old experiences, for example a sore joint
from a recent injury or a chronic stomach ache.

Tracking the body's sensations effectively pulls the
client into present time, rather than the traumatic past or the
anxiety-inducing future. When the physical body is observed

Body-Low-Slow-Loop Summary

Body

- Direct the attention into the body to notice a sensation.
- *This effectively means present-tense orientation, countering trauma's past-future tendency.*

Low

- Direct the attention to the lower border of the sensation, or downward generally.
- *This effectively counters the upward effect of trauma (alarm & orienting responses).*

Slow

- Ask about the details of the sensation.
- *This effectively slows down the awareness, countering trauma's tendency to speed things up.*

Loop

- Direct the attention somewhere else for a minute or so, then back to the first site. Repeat as needed, slowly and gently.
- *This effectively re-establishes polarized movement and counters trauma's tendency toward fixation.*

---

[36] Breath is particularly interesting because it is one of the few body functions with fully overlapping voluntary and involuntary control, an always-present interface between the conscious mind and the ANS. This partially accounts for attention to breathing as such a popular medi-tation and self-healing application.

in this mindful way, its unique processing capabilities are heightened. Instead of thinking about dire consequences or being buffeted by strong emotions, a client learns to convert awareness to a simple curiosity about the physicality of the experience. By shifting the attention to the more manageable physical level, the problematic emotional and mental dimensions may be temporarily set aside.

Low

Next, attention is directed downward to the lower border of the area being considered in Step One, or the southern body areas, such as feet or seat. This could consist of focusing on the lower edge of a problematic area or noticing the body's contact with the chair or floor. It does not need to be forced; if curiosity does not naturally lead to a lower perceptual target, we can just move on to the next step.

When we are startled or afraid, the body tends to elevate our center of gravity, for a host of physiological reasons, including heightened sensory sensitivity in the head, protection of peripheral limbs by reducing the circulation and activation of some of the most powerful stress response tools in the heart and brain. Guiding the attention downward effectively counters this upward effect of stress or fear.

Slow

The third step is to inquire about the details of the sensation. Detailed questions are posed, such as, "Is this more on the left or the right?" "Is it shallow or deep?" "Is it moving or still?" "Is it hard or soft?" There is no limit to the variety of these questions. The purpose is not about getting the information; it is about what happens when detailed questions are asked. The client could be guided to detect the texture of clothing, the temperature in the room, the border of the sensation or any number of focusing possibilities. One possibility is to ask the client to imagine having a felt-tip marker, and to visualize using it to trace the border of the body area that has become the focus of attention due to sensations. Another possibility is to ask the client to compare one side of the target area to the other side.

Often clients will use their hand to indicate which body area is generating the feeling or sensation. I have found that it is better to have them point to the area but not actually touch it. Touching can introduce new, different sensations and alter the natural awareness process.

Detailed questions cause our awareness to become more specific. When clients are asked these kinds of questions, they invariably pause, to try to figure out an answer. Their curiosity about their own sensation is heightened, causing a corresponding transfer of attention away from mental or emotional processes that may be overwhelming. Curiosity is a gesture of witness consciousness, automatically pulling us away from fixation.

Stress and trauma are notorious for their time-bending effects; time seems to speed up under stress. This step effectively slows down awareness processing, countering trauma's tendency to accelerate. By holding a curiosity about the sensation's specific attributes, the whole system starts to slow down.

Loop

The final step is derived from the great innovation developed by Peter Levine.[37] In the Loop phase, the client is directed to shift the attention somewhere else for a minute or so, then back to the first site. This is repeated once or twice as needed, slowly and gently. The key is to induce perceptual movement from pole to pole, a form of "That" (initial foreground sensation) and "Not That" (elsewhere in the body). Any second location can do the trick: noticing the feet or hands is a common choice because they are rarely the site of ANS activation, unless they were the main site of an injury.

[37] Levine, Peter. *In an Unspoken Voice.*

Under attack, we would naturally use our hands and feet to protect our more vulnerable torso and face, so the ANS seems to consider them to be less mission-critical or worthy of priority attention.

If the first area of attention has been uncomfortable or activated in any way, it is better to find a second site that is not experiencing unpleasant sensations, to establish a pole-to-pole process. The Loop part of BLSL sets up a temporary dipole in the awareness to facilitate or induce movement.

If clients are in pain or feel overwhelmed, they may report that they can't find another place to use for the second target. For such occurrences, we can induce sensation by touching their feet or some other contact, thereby creating increased sensory activity while asking the client to report what can be noticed. When doing the practice without a facilitator, we can lightly move our fingertips or toes against each other or whatever other surface we are touching, to amplify sensory nerve stimulation and signaling.

After a minute or two of focusing on the second location, the attention is brought back to the first view of the body, whichever area was being focused upon, and we begin

---

"That and Not That"

A foundation of perception is differentiation. In BLSL, the phrase "That and Not That" is shorthand for shifting sensory attention from one target to another. The focus is not so important as the shifting back and forth. Generally the various dimensions of the body are useful (top-bottom, left-right, front-back, core-periphery). Frequently "that" is a part that hurts in some way, and "not that" is another part that does not hurt.

In a larger sense, "That and Not That" means the action of a pendulum or recurrent feedback loop, in any form. Self-Other, Present-Past, Speaker-Listener are all examples. Pendulation is a key part of Somatic Experiencing, as it slowly undoes the body's tendency to fixate under the influence of trauma and stress.

---

again at the start of the Body-Low-Slow-Loop process. The first locale is often different, perhaps more diffuse, less painful or entirely uninteresting, due to the effect of restoring awareness movement.

Levine describes how dwelling for too long on a painful sensation or situation can deepen the problem, making us become more fixed in whatever painful state was initially created by the response to an incident. The Loop phase of the BLSL process effectively re-establishes pole-to-pole movement (a key tenant of Polarity Therapy) and counters trauma's tendency toward fixation.

Using BLSL as a Supportive Practice for Health

The BLSL practice can be done without any particular context or specific pain being present. Once a person has become familiar with it in stress-free times, it can be used when there is an upsetting situation, compulsion of any kind, heightened emotions such as fear or anger or other such ANS situations. Consistent practice seems to gradually strengthen autonomic functioning, as if the non-cognitive intelligence begins to trust that beneficial movement is the new normal, instead of harmful fixation. Research in neuroscience has clearly demonstrated that repetition can lead to the formation of new neural circuits; as a result, the benefits of BLSL repatterning could be long-lasting.

For example, a female client who was extremely fearful about air travel was encouraged to try Body-Low-Slow-Loop starting about eight weeks before an unavoidable trip, at least once daily for about fifteen minutes at a time. After the first two weeks of practicing without imagining any particular context, she began to visualize going to the airport as a prelude to the practice. Then in the next two weeks, she imagined waiting at the gate, then in the next two weeks, walking onto the plane, continuously repeating the same BLSL sequence. In the sixth week, she actually got in her car and drove a few blocks toward the airport, then did the practice. By the time the actual trip arrived, there was very little fear left, and she was able to travel without complications. She also reported many other benefits, including a decrease in general anxiety, better sleep and increased patience.

Bedtime is a good time to practice BLSL, using contact with the sheets and blankets as a sensory stimulus. By settling the system down just before sleeping, we can optimize the restorative powers of dreamtime. A few minutes of BLSL before sleep may also help a person integrate the day's experiences and re-train stress responses. BLSL has also been used effectively as a remedy for insomnia.

Body-Low-Slow-Loop offers a simple practice that anyone can learn, and it can be quite transformative. However, it seems to be out of range for some clients. For example, those who are in a deep depression or state of parasympathetic shock. These clients seem to be unable to remember the practice, or to stay with it for very long. In these cases, they need someone to coach them through the process, reminding them, and even stimulating sensation (for example, by rubbing the feet) in order to create a second pole for oscillation of awareness. A BLSL audio recording has been created specifically for the benefit of these clients who need a boost to get started at home.[38]

In another example, a client who suffered an auto accident was having panic attacks when driving to work, to the point of considering resigning from work to avoid the commute. She learned the BLSL method and experienced relief very quickly. In addition to symptom relief, she gained the great benefit of feeling less trapped. Instead of feeling helpless if a surge of anxiety started to appear, she knew she had a method to cope with the situation, and her fear did not esca-

---

[38] Chitty, John. *Body-Low-Slow-Loop.* www.energyschool.com.

late as it had before. She kept her job and did not need further sessions.

Similarly, a high school student was having panic attacks and learned BLSL in one session. She applied it in class and felt a reduced urgency in her anxiety. She was able to avoid a host of impending negative consequences and had a full recovery, without the expense of additional sessions.

BLSL is not a substitute for full-scale trauma resolution therapy. It is a first-aid strategy that belongs in our toolkit with other methods. It is easy to learn for all ages, applicable in diverse circumstances, self-empowering and free of cost. It could be a useful part of training for anyone who is in a potentially traumatic professional environment, such as law enforcement or the military. In addition, it offers emergency caregivers such as medical staff, police, ambulance drivers and school health personnel a valuable tool to use in difficult situations where ANS disturbances are common.

88. Boundary Practice

In this practice, clients are instructed in a three-step process to imagine a surrounding shell that can protect them from intrusive events. Ideally this shell is about arm's length from the body, in all directions, forming an invisible egg shape that defines an energetic boundary. The concept is similar to artists' depictions of the human aura. The boundary practice is another example of a mind-body healing interchange between conscious and subconscious processes: we consciously go through the practice, and repetitively doing it subtly changes our subconscious reality.

The boundary shell is analogous to the function of the immune system, which protects the inside of the body from the outside environment. Boundary-challenged individuals may be considered to have a weakened ANS and immune system, and the boundary practice can be a general remedy when we feel susceptible to upsets from outside ourselves, such as with other people who are irritating or threatening us in some way.

Three Steps: Inspect, Repair and Rest

The first step is to imagine and visualize a shell surrounding the whole body and to mentally examine its condition. Clients often report specific observations when they do this for the first time, such as having a boundary that is too close, missing in some areas, discolored or damaged; the imagined right-front-upper area may be quite different from the left-rear-lower area. The location of the boundary problem may have some relationship to real events in the past (for example a car accident from the left may come into memory when the left side is imagined), but the focus here is not on events. Here the boundary visualization is our present-time sensing process, unrelated to any one specific context.

In Step One, we sweep our attention from front-center to right, then right to rear, then rear to left, then left to front, forming an imaginal sense about the condition of the boundary or shell. Some areas may seem missing entirely, fragmented, too close, too far or any other variation.

In Step Two, we scan again, using the findings from Step One to imagine repairing the boundary in each quadrant. Any imaginary repair materials can be used: plaster, plexiglass, bricks and wood have all been conjured up by clients. The circular sweep of all four quadrants is conducted again, doing the repairs (in the imagination) as needed. The repair can also include re-setting the distance of the boundary, pushing it further out if it is too close and pulling it in if it is too far, with the intent to create a uniform distance from the body. There can be an imagined fortification of the shell, or a change in its color or texture. It can be imagined to have changed from opaque to transparent, so that approaching events can be seen. At the end of Step Two, we should be able to imagine a complete shell, with no holes or cracks, all at a consistent distance from the body. Far-fetched though it may seem, clients usually manage to create a sense of boundary repair.

Step Three is taking time to settle and rest within the newly restored boundary, feeling the effect of having our own secure, protected space. Within the shell, we have full choice about all interactions; no one else can enter without permission. This settling phase can be enjoyed for an extended period of time. Having a restored boundary can be quite a novelty for a person with chronic anxiety.

Some people have very disturbed boundaries, especially as echoes of early childhood when there may have been a high level of helplessness and intrusion. The boundary practice is extra useful for these people, but more repetition may be needed to really arrive at a felt sense of safety and protection within the energetic shield. It takes time and repetition for the felt sense of safety to become familiar and then habitual. Once again we are attempting to take advantage of how repetitive thought processes can re-wire the brain, in this case to a state of feeling safe.

In a variation of the practice, to make it more tangible, the client can sit on the floor and rolled blankets or towels can be placed in a surrounding circle, representing the boundary's ideal distance.

Part Three
Body Reading

"A person's past is his body."
                                        -- Lowen, *Bioenergetics*, p. 34.

"To every emotional state corresponds a personal conditioned pattern of muscular contraction, without which it [the emotional state] has no existence."
                    -- Feldenkrais, *Body and Mature Behavior*, p. 93.

"Now we know that the mind and body are like parallel Universes. Anything that happens in the mental universe must leave tracks in the physical one. As you see it right now, your body is the physical picture, in 3-D, of what you are thinking."
                                -- Chopra, *Quantum Healing*, p. 69.

Appreciating the link between physical, emotional and mental levels of our being is absolutely essential to understanding the energy approach to health. This section presents Polarity Therapy's approach to making the link direct and tangible.

For most people, pain is felt physically. Some are sensitive to emotional pain, but it is more subtle, as we do not have the sensory equipment to perceive it so directly. Mental pain is most subtle of all: while many may feel vague distress, only a few can recognize specifically when an unrealistic expectation or unworkable attitude is causing problems. We feel a splinter in the finger quite directly; an emotional splinter or hurt feelings, or a flaw in the mental blueprint, is much more difficult to perceive.

Body reading is a primary tool for energy practitioners. It provides information to serve many purposes, from identifying current and future health event probabilities, to linking the obvious symptom (in the physical body) with the subtle cause (in the emotions and mental patterns).

The whole notion of body reading is a revolutionary idea in the health field, and often difficult for the conventional practitioner to accept.

> Giving a physical foundation for psychiatry... was also a new concept. (Stone, *Polarity Therapy Vol. 1.* Book 1, p. 8)

> The first premise... is to assume that all movements of the body have meaning... I find this... most difficult to accept.[39]

Body reading is best used as a gentle indicator, rather than hard fact, and its goal primarily the prompting of self-understanding, not the diagnosis of disease.

In the Asia, body reading has a far more elevated place. Virtually all health systems from the East use some form of body reading: pulse diagnosis, physiognomy (reading the face), analysis of the eye, the ear, breath, voice quality, the torso, the hands and feet. In some cases these are very difficult for the Westerner to penetrate: Chinese pulse diagnosis in particular requires an intuitive sensitivity that eludes most western practitioners. Stone mentions that ancient Chinese pulse diagnosis distinguished over 600 different pulse qualities, far too complex for the newcomer to find useful.

> The Chinese physician can detect imbalances in meridians by feeling the pulses, but this is a sensi-

---

[39] Fast, Julius. *Body Language*. p. 151. This was one of the first popular books on the subject of body reading.

tive touch, and it may take 10 to 20 years to develop proficiency with it.[40]

Stone's Polarity Therapy made extensive use of body reading, and in a way that is relatively easy to understand. His system is based on the Ayurvedic system of India, although it is generally confirmed and supported by other systems which have made it to the West, such as Macrobiotics and Shiatsu.

There is a problem in the fact that body reading systems and techniques from Asia do not necessarily agree entirely with each other. This makes the study of body reading less tidy, and less valid for some: theoretically, if the information was accurate, all systems would say exactly the same thing, which they do not. Our recommendation is to proceed with caution and sincere curiosity, using experience as the primary validating procedure and emphasizing open-minded sensitivity in applying abstract ideas to individual cases.

> Information does not become knowledge unless it has relevance to experience... Knowledge becomes understanding when it is coupled with feeling.[41]

The energy practitioner is like a detective, searching for clues which could explain events. There are many sources for clues, and body reading is one of the best.

Replicated Patterns

The basis for Polarity body reading is thinking of the different areas (face, torso, hands and feet) as replicated patterns of a single design. The key to the design is the arrangement of energy zones, centers and fields along the spine, with their increasingly dense vibrations, located in a vertical order.

---

[40] Thie, John. *Touch for Health*. p. 17. He continues: "Touch for Health uses muscle testing to detect these same imbalances, taking advantage of the body's own wisdom to let us know what's going on."

[41] Lowen, Alexander. *Bioenergetics*. p. 62.

This is the Caduceus. We have discussed this idea of repeating patterns earlier with Babbitt's Atom and Reflexology.

What do we look for when beginning body reading from a Polarity perspective? There are two groups of questions for the beginner to ask: comparison of symmetries, to assess Three Principles (left/right, top/bottom and back/front), and analysis of horizontal-zones (of marks, swellings, lines or deviations from the norm), to assess the Five Elements. More advanced practitioners will look for more subtle cues, including more sophisticated views of top/bottom symmetry, front/back balance, posture (especially hips and shoulders) and others.

The two beginning questions (comparison of symmetries and location of marks) can be applied to any part of the body, but the face, torso and feet seem to be most immediately useful.

Symmetry

Very few people have symmetrical bodies. One side will be smaller, as measured on the face from the bottom of the eye to the corner of the mouth, or on the torso from shoulder to hip. The short side shows where tension originates, and more subtly, the aspect of experience that causes more stress. The right side suggests the condition of the Yang energy, the ease of Yang (creative, responsible, outgoing, logical, giving direction) for the individual, and the contribution of the father. The left side indicates the ease of Yin experience (receptive, yielding, intuitive, listening) for the person, and the contribution of the mother.[42] Which side is contracted? That will

---

[42] "...the left is the side with which we take things in. It is receptive. The right side is outgoing, expressive, the side with which we act." (Kurtz and Prestera, *The Body Reveals*, p. 47). Stone (*Polarity Therapy, Vol. 1*, Book 3, p. 29) and Dychtwald (*Bodymind*, p. 27) both agree with this.

be the aspect of life and parental mind-pattern of greatest stress.

Horizontal Energy Zones

Second, survey the area for marks and distortions. Which zone is disproportionately expanded or contracted? Where are the lines and bumps, how is makeup or jewelry used, where are scars or injuries? Into which of the five horizontal zones do these fall? According to theory, these are not accidental, but consistent with the overall subtle energy field of the individual.

This last statement is controversial for some, and requires a digression. Is there such a thing as a true accident or random event? Commonly used language suggests that there is, but deeper consideration suggests not.

> Life is from within out. External trauma and effects are in the fields of the external nature, of mechanical skill and principles. But the within rules the without. All external happenings are precipitated by unperceived, internal (mental- emotional) causes. (Stone, *Polarity Therapy Vol. 1.* Book 3, p. 35)

It is a central premise of this system that all events have a place in the cosmic plan. From our limited perspective we cannot see or comprehend the whole picture. Our quest is to discover those parts and patterns which can be known, and to make use of information gathered to increase knowledge and harmony. With body reading, we assume that all shapes, lines and events have a significance, even though we are limited in our understanding of the meaning.

Yin and Yang

The words Yin and Yang in this context refer to the ideas eloquently summarized in the *I Ching*.[43] It is important to note that Stone did not elaborate deeply on emotions or family patterns in his therapy, and as we move into this area, we are no longer fully supported by his writings. His use of the words Yin and Yang focused primarily on the electromagnetic attributes of the basic polarity relationships in nature. Here we add a much wider range of psychological interpretation.

Generally, Yang refers to outgoing experience, our impulse to be, to act and to do in the world. It is manifested in breath as inhalation and (usually) in brain function by the left hemisphere activities. We all must act on our impulses, and ultimately face the challenge of being responsible (or able to respond) to the results of those actions. Yang also refers to the masculine aspect of experience, which is steady, logical and aggressively goal oriented. Qualities of Yang are represented by the sperm, its purest manifestation. Yang is also the centrifugal direction of involutionary movement: flowing outward from its source, Yang is the soul's pathway into the material world.

Complementarily, Yin refers to the incoming experience, our receiving of impulses from outside ourselves. It is manifested in breath as exhalation, in blood flow as veins, and (usually) in brain function by the right hemisphere activities. We all struggle to deal with external events, and we all must

---

[43] Wilhelm, Richard, translator. *I Ching.* p. 3-15. This section describes the extension of the ideas of Yin and Yang into many aspects of human experience. For a summary from an East Asian expert: "The principles of Yin and Yang are: 1) All things have two aspects, a Yin aspect and a Yang aspect; 2) A Yin or Yang aspect can be further divided into Yin and Yang; 3) Yin and Yang mutually create each other; 4) Yin and Yang control each other; and, 5) Yin and Yang transform into each other." – Kaptchuk, Michael. *The Web That Has No Weaver.* p. 7-12.

ultimately face the challenge of accepting what comes to us. Yin also refers to the feminine aspect of experience, for men or women, which is cyclic, intuitive, absorbing and pulling. Qualities of Yin are represented by the egg, its purest manifestation. Yin is also the centripetal direction of evolutionary movement: having landed in matter, Yin is the soul's pathway back toward spirit.

Linkage of Yang/right side with father and Yin/left side with mother is hinted in Stone's writings, and is clearly expressed elsewhere.

> We associate the left side of the body (which is controlled primarily by the right side of the brain) with feelings, emotions, and the relations to the mother. The right side is associated with the father, reason, thinking, logic.[44]

These ideas of Yin and Yang have a tremendous universality, and are useful for psychological inquiry. In the Asia, it is said that there are only four diseases, too much or too little of the two basic modes of energy flow. In the dysfunctional relationships model of modern psychology represented by Virginia Satir and others, these four are found as archetypes: the tyrant (too much Yang), wimp (too little Yang), doormat (too much Yin) and critic (too little Yin). Relationships tend to represent magnetic equality, with too much or too little being inevitably, magnetically drawn to each other in magnetically powerful, but destructive, painful and unstable relationships.

Before we begin the body reading of specific areas, two of Stone's relevant charts are provided for general reference. The first, known as Weaving the Body, provides basic information about relationships of the Three Principles and Five Elements. The second, 25 Combinations, gives a key for linking the Five Elements with emotions.

---

[44] Kurtz and Prestera. *The Body Reveals*. p. 47. See also pages 97-100.

Weaving the Body

Source: *Polarity Therapy Vol. 1*, Book 1, p. 48-53

Weaving the Body

In the chart on the preceding page, the language of astrology is used to convey subtle physical, emotional and mental relationships that are relevant for energy-based body reading. Stone was careful to emphasize that his use of astrology was for its useful archetypal language, and not for what he called "divination," or trying to tell the future.

Languages are filters by which we make sense of input, through categorizing experience into recognizable, meaningful systems. Language has great power, the medium becoming the message. Expectations about people and objects are formed according to the language used to name and describe them.

The simplest language is Yes/No, or That/Not That. Yes/No reflects the fundamental reality of human experience, i.e., approach for reward or pull back from threat. Yes/No divides experience by two, the smallest possible divisor. Yang/Yin is just such a duality language. The naming of objects and events occurs on this simple yes/no level: giving something a name makes it distinct from its surroundings: "that" and "not that."

More sophisticated languages divide by larger factors: to categorize by three leads to the Three Principles, by four leads to the four seasons, directions, and classic Elements. Twelve (Zodiac, clock, calendar) is particularly useful, since it neatly incorporates two, three and four. Twelve-part Astrology language unifies the ideas of Yang/Yin, the Three Principles and the four lower Elements into a single system: each sign is a unique mix of these three factors.

As examples of larger systems, ten (numbers), 26 (alphabet), 64 (*I Ching* hexagrams) show how even more complex filters have been developed to describe human experience.

There is also a quest for no division at all, or oneness. This is a state of mind associated with deep spiritual experience. At this level, no language can function. Mystic traditions speak of a level of awareness beyond language in which man realizes and merges with Unity, in the "Peace which passeth all understanding."

25 Combinations:
Weaving the Body with the Five Elements

Source: *Polarity Therapy Vol. 2.* p. 226-227.

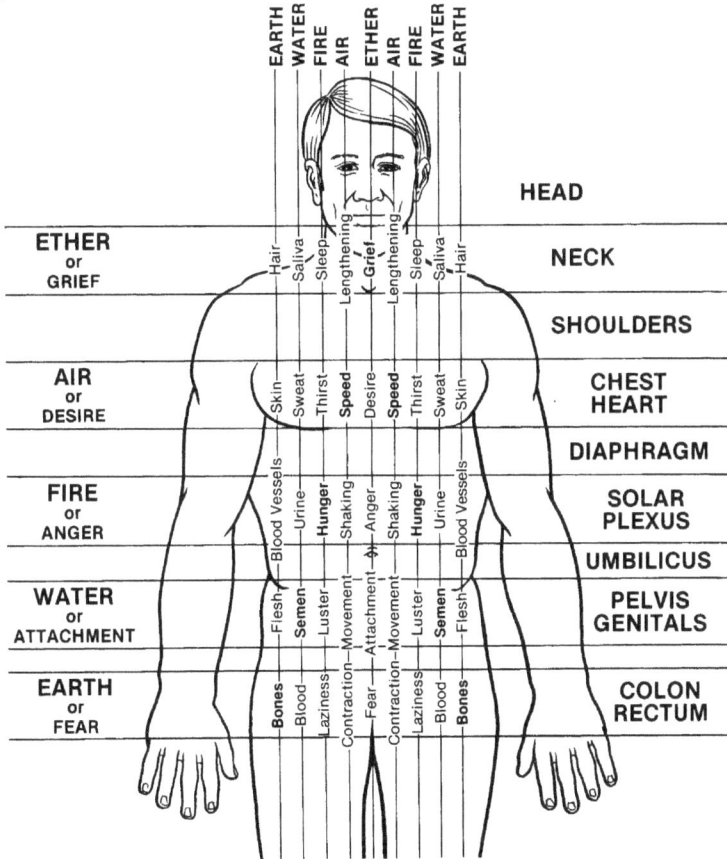

EARTH
WATER
FIRE
AIR
ETHER
AIR
FIRE
WATER
EARTH

HEAD

ETHER
or
GRIEF

NECK

Hair—Saliva—Sleep—Lengthening—**Grief**—Lengthening—Sleep—Saliva—Hair

SHOULDERS

AIR
or
DESIRE

CHEST
HEART

Skin—Sweat—Thirst—**Speed**—Desire—**Speed**—Thirst—Sweat—Skin

DIAPHRAGM

FIRE
or
ANGER

SOLAR
PLEXUS

Blood Vessels—Urine—**Hunger**—Shaking—Anger—Shaking—**Hunger**—Urine—Blood Vessels

UMBILICUS

WATER
or
ATTACHMENT

PELVIS
GENITALS

Flesh—**Semen**—Luster—Movement—Contraction—Attachment—Contraction—Movement—Luster—**Semen**—Flesh

EARTH
or
FEAR

COLON
RECTUM

Bones—Blood—Laziness—Contraction—Fear—Contraction—Laziness—Blood—Bones

This diagram is a summary of Stone's "Enquiry into the Gross Body" charts, which are in turn derived from ancient Indian sources. The center line shows the emotions for each elemental zone. This is the basis for Polarity Therapy's linking of body and emotions, a major topic in body reading.

Body Reading for the Face

Of all the parts of the body, none is so directly expressive of a person as that complex unity of structure we call a face.[45]

To analyze the face at an introductory level, we apply the same left/right and horizontal zones approaches. The left/right comparison may be facilitated by covering one side, then the other. Which side is contracted, as measured from corner of the mouth to the eye? Does one side convey a specific feeling more than the other? An interesting study is to use a popular magazine, one with many pictures, and apply this idea to many faces chosen randomly. Very few faces will be symmetrical, and the emotions expressed can be dramatic when one side is covered.

The horizontal zones may be viewed generally or individually. Generally, what is the overall image? Which zone seems most stressed? Stress is indicated by marks, scars, discoloration, loss of tone, creases or other unusual signs.

For specific zones, we begin at the top. The area from the cheeks up indicates the Air Element, in the chest. The eyebrows reflect the shoulders and the upper cheek the breast/lung area. Dark circles under the eyes mean kidney stress, the kidneys being the neutral pole of the Air Element as shown on the "Weaving the Body" chart. Air is manifested emotionally as desire, as shown on the "25 Combinations" chart, including hope and ambition. Thus indicators in these areas of the face suggest desire (including hope or hopelessness) as an active source of stress.

Lower, across the nose and including the lower cheeks and the area above the mouth, is the zone for Fire Element, in the solar plexus. The lines from the nostrils around the mouth

---

[45] Kurtz and Prestera, *The Body Reveals*, p. 89

reflect the line of the diaphragm in the center of the Fire area. The nostrils and tip of the nose are heart indicators. Emotionally unbalanced or stressed fire manifests as anger or emotional coldness, so deep lines or a swollen nose suggest these as active emotional issues. Conversely, contraction here is a sign of constriction of power and capacity for love.

The mouth area and upper jaw area reflect the status of the Water Element, in the pelvis. The lips show the condition of the lower abdominal and genital area, with the upper lip related to Yang (outgoing, paternal) and lower lip related to Yin (receiving, maternal). The tip of the tongue also indicates sexuality and genital condition. These may be observed closely when bodywork or emotional process work is underway, to indicate activation of old emotions relating to attachment or sexuality. The lower cheeks or jowls indicate tone of the pelvic floor area. The emotion related to water is attachment or clinging, so these indicators show the degree to which attachment is a source of tension.

Identification of the lips and tip of the tongue as genital reflexes is a topic which has been described in several sources. Michio Kushi describes kissing as an unconscious electromagnetic surrogate for intercourse through reflex action. Similarly, painting the lips bright colors makes sense as a use of subliminal reflexology to stimulate sexual interest. This

The first two questions for Face Reading
Left/Right: Which side is more contracted?
Zones: Which zone has distortions, marks or expressive emphasis?

leads into other topics, such as the interpretation of other make-up practices (blue and green on the eyes being the colors for Ether and Air, or loneliness and desire, red on the cheeks as a reflex to the breast, etc.), and the many behaviors based on unconscious reflex perceptions.

The Earth area at the base of the spine is seen in the lower chin and jaw line. Lines and marks here suggest tension relating to fear, the emotion manifesting from the Earth Element. Look for marks, loss of tone, different skin color and other cues for distress in this zone.

Putting these observations of the face together with our earlier left/right comparison, we can offer a few guesses about the individual. Which element (and therefore emotion) is indicated, and in which style or from what parent? Which areas in the torso are likely to be involved?

In therapy, the practitioner watches the client's face closely. Movements and gestures can be subtle and easily missed. The face reflects current-time activity and is invaluable as a window on inner experience.

As a final comment on body reading for the face, the eyes need special attention. This is outside the left/right and horizontal zone analyses, and not derived primarily from Stone's writing. Stone's commentary on the eyes identifies them as the positive poles of the Yang Principle, "to give external direction for the internal impulses." (Stone, *Polarity Therapy Vol. 1*. p. 77) More recent research has provided more information on this. Observing the eyes shows which part of the brain is activated, how the person processes information and the level of stress present.[46]

----

[46] References for eye movement's relation to brain activity include: Robbins, Dennison, Stokes and Whiteside. Reading the eyes is a major specialty in body reading, giving quick and accurate information about unconscious or hidden feelings and brain function. This area is well worth detailed exploration for energy-based health practitioners.

"Sanpaku" is a Japanese term meaning "three whites," a condition in which white is visible below the iris (eye is rolled up, a Yin condition) or above the iris (eye is rolled down, a Yang condition). Either of these shows serious imbalance; extreme Sanpaku indicates danger to life (Yin being danger to self, Yang being danger to others). Sanpaku also changes with age, as the eye moves from Yang to Yin position (Yang at the start in newborns, Yin at the end in death).

Flickering or twitches of the eyes, and poor eyesight suggest imbalance (excess or deficiency) of Yang energy. If on the right, it indicates stress relating to applying force and creativity to a situation and, more remotely, to Father. If on the left, it suggests stress relating to receiving creative energy or authority, and Mother.

Body Reading for the Torso

Reading the language of the torso repeats the basic approach described for the face. However the torso also has additional variables including posture, breathing and expressive movements. Comparable ways of body reading exist for the face, but they are very subtle. With the torso, they become more obvious.

One of the best ways to access this information is to mimic the person being studied.

> If one assumes the bodily attitude of another person, one can sense the meaning, have the feeling of, that body expression.[47]

Twenty years later this technique would become known as "matching" in Neuro-Linguistic Programming (NLP), used for diagnosis and also as a way of influencing people.

The general guiding concept of looking at the right side for Yang indicators, and the left for Yin, continues to apply. In the torso, which hip is higher? Usually, the high hip indicates

---

[47] Feldenkrais, Moshe. *Body and Mature Behavior.* p. 93.

the side which has greater stress. Similarly, which shoulder is lower? Look along the diaphragm area for signs of contraction, swelling or rigidity. Look for scars left by accidents or surgeries. Which side are they on?

The idea of horizontal zones for each element, and of elements being associated with specific emotions, can be applied again: look at each horizontal zone and characterize its appearance with a few words. Is it expanded or contracted? What is the tone of skin and muscles? Are there unusual marks or distortions? Are there scars or injuries?

Then, refer to the "25 Combinations" chart to know what emotion relates to the area. With this information, formulate a hypothesis which combines the descriptive words with the relevant emotions, possibly also in terms of Yang (right side) or Yin (left side). You are now using the simplest level of body reading!

For example, a caved in chest (Air) can reflect sunken hopes and lost desire. A rigid or swollen solar plexus (Fire) can indicate withheld or chronically present anger. A swollen pelvis (Water) can suggest excessive enmeshment and holding on. Tightened buttocks with locked knees, and tight walk (Earth) could reflect chronic anxiety or fear.

After learning these basic ideas for torso body reading, combine them with the earlier discussion of the face. A good way to do this is to look in a mirror at your own face. Look for right/left differences. Which side is more contracted? Then, look at the horizontal bands of air, fire, water and earth: are any of these disproportionately large (expanded) or small (contracted)? Are there any marks or distortions?

With your observations for the face complete, look at the torso. Follow the same sequence, looking for left/right comparisons first, then horizontal zones. Do you notice any correlations between face and torso?

Body reading for the torso requires a more inclusive, general perspective, observing the overall body. This con-

Torso/Foot Reflexology Relationships
The torso organs, spine and foot are related energetically,
as shown in this overlay view.

trasts with the specific focus used with the face. In addition to
the left/right and horizontal zone analysis described for the
face, the whole person is considered. Robbins identifies eight
main areas to watch in body reading: breathing, eye movement, lower lip size, posture, muscle tone and pupil. Our experience has tended to emphasize four of these: breathing,
eye movement, posture and voice are easily available, accu-

rate signals well worth study.[48] We also add hand gestures to the list in the following introduction to these specialized subjects.

Breathing indicates the measure of participation in life, and whether a person is holding back (over- or under-expansion, a Yang imbalance) or holding on (over- or under-contraction, a Yin imbalance). Some successful therapies, including Reichian psychiatry, Re-birthing, and Kundalini Yoga, begin and in some cases dwell entirely on the expansion and balancing of breath.

Posture is a major area. The unique upright stance of man allows a delicate blending of gravitational response and subtle moving toward vs. moving away from positioning, which expresses a person's psychological attitude. This is developed with great detail by Feldenkrais and Keleman. The use of the arms and hands, the carriage of the shoulders, spine and pelvis, the style of gait and postural response to stimulation of various kinds can all be interpreted valuably.

Lowen classifies posture in two general categories which mesh perfectly with Polarity theory. He characterizes mankind as having two general styles of motivation, aggression (to push, Yang) and longing (to pull, Yin). He found a direct reflection in the spine: those too insecure to act (Yang imbalance) had locked knees and rigid pelvis; those unable to receive life's pressures with successful adaptation and emotional processing (Yin imbalance) had rounded shoulders and a slumping neck, the "dowager's hump."[49]

This idea has been developed further by Keleman. Building on the theme of the duality of pulsation (expansion and contraction, or Yang and Yin) he shows a continuum of postural change from resistance to exhaustion, from youthful ambition to elderly fatigue.

---

[48] Robbins, Tony. *Unlimited Power.* p. 328.

[49] Lowen, Alexander. *BioEnergetics.* pp. 236, 250, 299.

Hand placement is an important part of postural body reading. The hands will move naturally to the zones whose emotions are activated, either to suppress or release expression. When the hands are crossed over the solar plexus, a diaphragm stress (Fire/anger) is indicated; when touching the hips (Water), enmeshment/clinging or abandonment is communicated; when touching the mouth, sexuality and clinging; when at the throat, expression or grief, etc. Often you can intuitively gain insight into the activated element by replicating the posture, especially with the hands.

Voice is similar to eyes. You can differentiate qualities of sound by tone and loudness. Lower tones indicate lower elements, greater loudness suggests more Yang. Furthermore, important cues for identifying elements involved can be found in pitch, speed and timbre: Beaulieu and Robbins, among others, offer detail in this area.

Lowen emphasizes the therapeutic significance of voice quality:

> If a person is to recover his full potential for self-expression, it is important he gain the full use of his voice in all its registers and in all its nuances of feeling.[50]

Many other levels are possible; we recommend using the references cited to pursue the subject.[51]

Among many possibilities, this observation supports the idea of singing being beneficial for emotional wellness.

As we have seen, the assignment of emotional qualities to specific body areas is one of the great contributions of Stone to body reading. This idea of identifying the emotion and therefore the mental process behind illnesses according to

---

[50] Lowen, Alexander. *BioEnergetics*. p. 271.

[51] For psychological body reading, recommended sources are: Stokes and Whiteside (*Under the Code* and *One Brain*), LaBorde (*Influencing with Integrity*), Hay (*Heal Your Body*) and Dychtwald (*Bodymind*).

the location of the problem has also been advanced by others. Louise Hay's *Heal Your Body,* which gives very specific identifications, is a notable example.

Body Reading for the Feet

The following material on body reading for the feet is somewhat removed from Randolph Stone. There are Polarity references supporting some of this section's conclusions (identifying the toes as relating to specific chakras, identifying specific emotions relating to those chakras, and linking Yang or masculine energy with the right foot, and Yin, or feminine energy, with the left). But the larger psychological interpretations presented here are not found directly in Stone's writing.

We offer these ideas in a spirit of experimentation, for practitioners to use and validate for themselves. There is no scientific data or research to support these theories. All we have to go on is a wealth of anecdotal experience, and we invite readers to approach the topic in that light.

Our theory has three parts, which will each be discussed separately:

1. That the shape of the toe indicates the chronic condition of the corresponding energy center.

2. That the energy center, as exhibited by the shape of the toe, can be analyzed directly in terms of its etheric manifestation, or emotion.

3. That the left and right feet reflect a person's sensory experience of Yin and Yang energies, and that these energies generally reflect the blueprint contribution of mother and father, respectively.

1. The shape of the toe indicates the chronic condition of the corresponding energy center.

Correspondences are depicted by Stone showing Earth, Water, Fire, Air, and Ether centers represented by toes in order from small to large.

In this context, "shape" means tone (circulation, flexibility, presence of callous or bunion), alignment (location, direction, whether one toe is parallel to other toes) and symmetry (size and shape compared to other toes). "Chronic" in this situation refers to long-term family patterns inherited both genetically and emotionally.

> These living current areas divide the body into five zones or fields of receptivity, like the use of the five senses over the five fingers and toes on each side of the body, over which they actually flow. This is a vertical classification of areas of response of the five energy currents operating in the body. (Stone, *Polarity Therapy Vol. 2.* p. 33)

> The bones and the joints of the fingers and toes often give a hint in diagnosis, where everything else is obscure and indefinite, and the patient merely exists and suffers. This is nature's own finger of diagnosis and indication, and not mere theory. It reveals the disrupted relationship of the extremities on the surface with the centers of energy within, in the particular region specified by the finger or toe. (Stone, *Polarity Therapy Vol. 1.* Book 3, p. 39)

> Precipitation occurs most often here [the foot] because of its great distance from the invigorating center. (Stone, *Polarity Therapy Vol. 1.* Book 3, p. 38)

2. The energy center, as expressed by the shape of the toe, can be analyzed directly in terms of its etheric manifestation, or emotion.

> The body suffers as an innocent bystander, not as the causative factor. But it gets all the blame because effects and end products accumulate there as precipitates of highly emotional chemical action. (Stone, *Polarity Therapy Vol. 1.* Book 3, p. 35)

The emotions are identified by Stone in his "Enquiry into the Gross Body" charts, summarized as "25 Combinations" earlier. For our purposes, we focus on the center line of the illustration, in which an etheric component for each chakra is identified.

These emotions and chakras are: Earth/Fear, Water/ Attachment, Fire/Anger, Air/Desire, and Ether/Grief. This linkage of emotions and physical centers has enormous implications, for it supplies the seeker of self-understanding with a way to translate that which is obvious and physical, into that which is hidden and subtle. This is the missing link between physiology and psychology, one of the points of extraordinary genius about Polarity Therapy. The Polarity practitioner can be giving a session, touching a certain area, and observe the activation of the appropriate emotions.

With the knowledge contained in this chart, these emotions make sense, and can be processed in specific ways. Old feelings can be freed from their deep storage in the tissues, brought into consciousness, and comprehended as family patterns, deeply-held attitudes and emotional reactions. This comprehension is a liberating experience of tremendous significance, for in understanding does man gain access to the blueprint and power to change his life.

Without defusion of past causors, no present time correction lasts longer than the next stressor.[52]

Facing old emotional traumas, bravely experiencing denied or forgotten pain, maturely comprehending what happened, forgiving those who have created harm and letting go, is a sure avenue to profound health improvement.

3. The left and right feet reflect a person's sensory experience of Yin and Yang energies, and these energies generally reflect the blueprint contribution of mother and father, respectively.

---

[52] Stokes and Whiteside. *One Brain*. p 5.

This statement requires explanation at every stage of the sentence.

> This life pattern began by the energy current flow in the male spermatozoon and the female ovum center of vitelline jelly substance, like a thread in a shuttle which travels forward and backward to weave the most wonderful fabric of life, called the human body. The pattern of the body was supplied by the mental and vital energy of the parents, according to their kind and stature. Of course, heritage goes back much further than that, but this is the general rule.
> (Stone, *Polarity Therapy Vol. 1.* Book 1, p. 9)

The idea that the soles of left and right feet are considered to reflect Yin and Yang energies for the front, or sensory side of the body is illustrated by Stone in several places. Waves of electromagnetic current have specific direction, flowing down and out of the front of the right foot, and up and in the front of the left foot.

We are concerned with the sensory side (the front side of the body) because of its significance in processing emotions. The "five pointed star" is the field which receives the impulses from above, where "sensory tension and emotional frustration" are recorded and stored.

Toe Reading

Assuming that our three basic premises are understood and accepted for testing, how do we apply them? We begin with an abstract illustration, below. The right foot shows an ideal arrangement, in which the toes are in relative proportion and pointing straight to the front. The left foot has the Earth (smallest) toe out of line. According to our theory, this suggests chronic fear (the emotion corresponding to the Earth chakra) in the Yin aspect of experience.

The Polarity detective might use these clues to formulate an hypothesis: this person's stress has to do with Earth Element (fear) experience in childhood, in a Yin context. With this initial general clue, the detective can then proceed to a more informed search for specific information.

Polarity practitioners often observe the toes as they begin a session for insights and clues about how to proceed. Subtle underlying causes may be understood efficiently, and the energy currents can be restored to a more natural flow.

Toe Reading Examples

The alignment of the toes is a valuable way to understand the flow of energy in the body. Observe which toes are distorted, and analyze the distortion in the context of the whole foot. The samples above are illustrations of the method.

Body reading for the toes provides information for therapy or self-understanding, but it must be approached without pathological thinking. The shape of the toes serve as an optimistic reminder about life challenges, not a pessimistic outlook about conditions.

Yin Principle & Fire Element

Yang Principle & Water Element

Yang Principle & Earth Element;
Also Yin Principle & Ether Element

Yang Principle & Fire Element

Yang Principle & Air Element

Yang Principle & Water Element

Part Four
Essays

1. The Journey of the Soul

Polarity Therapy is profound in its rich blending of health and philosophy. In ancient times, the concerns of the scientist and philosopher were unified: in Stone's writing, the two move effortlessly together.

The essential questions at the heart of philosophical inquiry are, What is humanity? Why are we here? What is consciousness, and life? Stone's answers to these questions constitute "the Journey of the Soul," which is presented at the very beginning of his written work and forms the foundation for all that follows.

Here is a summary of the Journey of the Soul, in Stone's words.

> ...The soul which inhabits this body is a unit of consciousness from another sphere, of much finer essences... Each incarnating soul or entity brings with it a design of life, of its own, by which it differs from others... (Stone, *Polarity Therapy Vol. 1.* Book 1, p. 9)

> The soul... steps down its energy and becomes a slave of the mind, and expresses itself through the senses. The senses relate to the mind as units to the whole... seeking experience in multiplicity and outward expenditure of energy... In matter, it is action for the sake of action; namely, the sensations, the enjoyment of the senses, the reactions, the accumula-

tion of things and personal honor, pride and self-aggrandizement through possessions and power...
[but] Every pleasure in this world, indulged in as such, has its resulting sorrow- if not immediately, at some time in the future. The same principle is still active when a child insists on touching a hot stove; it must experience the sensation and the resulting pain. (Stone, *Polarity Therapy Vol. 1.* Book 1, p. 31)

Our energies are constantly going outward, seeking in things the thrills and satisfactions which are not there. It is a mirage. Only the very highest universal source really has what we seek and crave. So, after maturity of years, after aeons of wanderings and sufferings, the soul finally is convinced of this fact and, like the 'Prodigal Son', remembers his Father's house and all its abundance. He then rises up within himself, turns his energy and longings of the soul inwards, and comes back home to his Universal Source... (Stone, *Polarity Therapy Vol. 1.* Book 3, p. 29)

Stone thus describes life as a school, with a centrifugal force propelling units of consciousness out from a primordial source, into the dense world of experience (involution), until through painful experience the deepest lessons are learned, providing the motivation for a centripetal return to the center (evolution).

The purpose is for the experience of souls embodied in forms and placed in outer space of matter and resistance in order to gain awareness through perception and action, for the fulfillment of consciousness. (Stone, *Polarity Therapy Vol. 1.* Book 3, p. 11)

Man alone stands at the top of the ladder of all Creation. He alone is endowed with all the faculties necessary to understand his Source, his Being, and his relationship to Nature. Writings of the Ancients became sacred because they endeavored to reveal to man some hints about his Source, his marvelous pent-up energies and soul powers, and how to use them wisely in Nature, how to transcend the ego and thereby find his way to his REAL HOME. (Stone, *Health Building*, p. 23)

This world is the School of Life. We come to gain experience, and have these bodies for that purpose. Through painful "burning of fingers" we learn to transcend the ego (our illusory confusion of true self with senses, body and mind) and seek deeper meaning. Thus the art of Polarity Therapy becomes the art of self-realization, which ultimately is the same as the quest for God-realization. A health system merges seamlessly into a profound spiritual understanding and worldview that unifies the beliefs of the world's major religions.

-JC

2. Mind and Body

The inclusion of psychology in physical medicine is inevitable, as the atomic era proceeds. It would be well within Stone's predictions to reach a time when, along with the allopathic treatment saving the patient from his symptoms, the practitioner of the healing arts would routinely do more, by looking for the subtle causes of the problems.

In this more holistic future, practitioners would alert patients to the fact that something was not working in their lives, and nudge them gently back toward the path of self-discovery, in hopes of identifying unworkable mental attitudes, indigestible emotional experiences, and destructive physical habits. Patients, in their pain, thus acquire support for increased personal responsibility and personal growth.

Getting the flu... is like getting a news update.[53]

This discussion would not be complete without mention of limitation. The holistic approach to health has in the past been guilty of oversimplifying the cause and treatment of disease. Pelletier cautions eloquently against the "Calvinist" attitude that people have defects which are to blame for their problems.

> Books on holistic health like to say that sick people "need" their sickness. Mainstream psychiatry points its own finger when it says that chronic diseases stand symbolically for self-punishment, revenge, or a deep feeling of worthlessness. I will not argue these insights except to suggest that they may be harmful to the healing process rather than helpful. It is hard enough for any of us to face up to our emotional fallibility even at the best of times. Can we really be expected to reform when we are ill?[54]

[53] Pelletier, Kenneth. *Mind as Healer, Mind as Slayer.* p. 10.

[54] Chopra, Deepak. *Quantum Healing.* p. 158.

We can't know the whole story behind illness. As Stone said, "heritage goes back much further than that," (Stone, *Polarity Therapy Vol. 1*. Book 1, p. 9) and there are too many variables.

> Each incarnating soul or entity brings with it a design of life, of its own, by which it differs from others. (Stone, *Polarity Therapy Vol. 1*. Book 1, p. 9)

In addition to the knowable contributions of parents, culture, environment and other forces, there is always an unknown factor carried from previous forgotten experience. The concept of re-incarnation, of previous lifetimes leading to the present, is inevitable and well-supported by many sources.[55]

A middle ground is recommended, acknowledging "Whatever works, works!" (Stone's motto), and constantly seeking greater self-knowledge, tempering body reading with a humble realization that full understanding is impossible. We seek a balance between the idea of personal responsibility for disease, which presses for self-improvement, and acceptance of our limits in either knowing or being able to control our circumstances. Like polarized energy, either side is incomplete without the other. It is misleading, deluding and frustrating to hint that perfect, comprehensive knowledge can ever be gained, for it is beyond human vision and capability.

> Polarity Therapy is not based on the illusion that one can achieve a state of constant relaxation and an end to all conflicts. It is rather based on the fact that most people are capable of using their energies more effectively.[56]

This search for self knowledge can only be a middle way, combining responsible action (balanced Yang) and discriminating acceptance (balanced Yin), and a certain comfort

---

[55] For example, see Richard Gerber's *Vibrational Medicine*, p. 161 and p. 484.

[56] Arroyo, Stephen. *Astrology, Psychology and the Four Elements*. p. 182.

This metaphorical art by Mark Allison depicts the plight of the soul, torn between materialism and its Source. The Involutionary Yang experience links the soul to the mind (the chariot), which is in turn pulled by the senses (the animals). The Evolutionary Yin experience turns the soul's attention back toward its "True Home."

Further symbolism is given here for the five elements in their manifestation as negative emotions: Horse (Ether, Pride); Pig (Air, Greed); Crocodile, (Fire, Anger); Vulture, (Water, Attachment); Snake (Earth, Fear). The symbolism of the Sun as the true home, or God, is based on the Sanskrit term "Ha" which means sun, the primal Yang creative force.

with the limitation of the knowledge available. This attitude is consistent with the scientific basis for the Polarity model, best expressed as Heisenberg's Uncertainty Principle (we can know a particle's direction or velocity, but not both), which transformed the study of physics at the turn of the century.

In this context, it is quite fitting that Stone walked away from his blossoming inquiry into esoteric health, the worldly passion of his entire life, to spend his last seven years in an ashram in India, meditating on spiritual matters.

Unlimited possibilities are not suited to man; if they existed, his life would dissolve in the boundless.[57]

Thus his final teaching is to keep our worldly efforts in perspective. Ultimately, the entire truth is not to be known, and the personal inner quest for higher understanding is more important anyway.   -JC

[57] Wilhelm, Richard (translator). *I Ching.* p. 232.

3. Medical Politics

"The two medicines do not have to be antagonists, but for the moment they clearly face in opposite directions."[58]

"It is unfortunate that mainstream medicine still acts as if it believes the Newtonian concepts, that have been proven to be an inaccurate model for fifty years, are real."[59]

Energy-based health systems are often considered to be antithetical to conventional western medicine. In body reading, where we attempt to directly link physical qualities with emotional/mental factors, this potential conflict is brought to center stage, because the idea is so alien to the mechanical model.

The conventional separation of body from emotions and mind is understandable because of the difficulty and complexity of working with the more subtle factors. In the West, there is a long history of the development of treatments for the physical level, but only a short history for emotional or mental treatment, usually confined to emergency care based on chemical medication. Before Freud, there were few pioneers in the field, and the succeeding generation struggled against a variety of restraints.

Only in the last few decades has the field expanded rapidly, to eventually begin to reach the common person. There is a grass roots movement bringing these ideas into common knowledge, often entirely bypassing the conventional system. A sign of this is the popularity of the many "12 Step" programs. Alcoholics Anonymous and its offspring deserve great credit for bringing mental support to the public.

---

[58] Chopra, Deepak. *Quantum Healing*, p. 141.

[59] Norman Cousins, quoted in Richard Gerber's *Vibrational Medicine*, p. 27.

Physical events requiring medical attention receive treatment aimed primarily at saving the patient from life-threatening symptoms, and relieving pain. These are vital and worthy goals, essential to the quality of life. We are the beneficiaries of the removal of major diseases from our cultural landscape, achieved by this system.

The practitioner of the energy approach can supplement conventional care by helping a person look at the subtle issues involved in disease. No amount of reflexology, exercise or self-understanding will save a person from acute appendicitis; but once saved by drugs and surgery, a follow-up holistic program of health enhancement will invariably be beneficial. The energy practitioner can support emergency health providers by helping people understand themselves better, helping them see how health problems often originate in more subtle sources relating to diet, lifestyle, emotional experience or mental attitudes

Sadly, these preventative dimensions of public health have been neglected by modern medicine for a variety of reasons. At a time of ever-increasing health care costs, the very inexpensive, self-regulated techniques of the energy approach could be a great asset to national well-being.

We advocate a cooperative attitude between these two branches of the health care system. Juhan makes an eloquent plea for such cooperation.[60]

> Western medicine, which has largely to do with the diagnosis of disease and severe malfunction, knows precious little about exercise and other preventative systems. It is neither useless nor unintelligent, only incomplete.[61]

–JC

---

[60] Juhan, Deane, *Job's Body*, p. 56.

[61] Horwitz, Tem. *T'ai Chi Ch'uan*, p. 18.

4. How the Body Tells the Truth

A neurophysiological explanation of the truthfulness of body language is given by Stokes and Whiteside in *One Brain*. Two subdivisions of the brain are noted: between "dominant" and "alternate" halves (a left/right distinction) and between "conscious associational thinking" (CAT) and "common integrative areas" (CIA) (a front/back distinction). Generally, language skills reside in the dominant half, and physical expression resides in the alternate half. The frontal CAT area holds newly-acquired knowledge, while the rear CIA holds survival skills gained earlier in the development of the species. The CIA is located in the dominant brain; the CAT is found in both left and right halves.

The CAT has the ability to control all neurological activity. However, under stress we characteristically "retreat" from the more advanced front CAT area to the survival-oriented, risk-avoiding back CIA zone. With its strong link to the dominant verbal side, the CIA generates the words we use under stress. These words will tend to reflect an association of current sensation with unconscious remembered experience, which has been strongly modulated by expectations and social customs. So for people who are under stress, words tend to express what they think they should say (their habitual pain-avoidance strategies) rather than how they actually feel.

Meanwhile the physical expression function in the alternate brain freely responds to the current sensation directly and independently. Thus the body language message will be simpler, clearer and more present-oriented than the verbal message, and much more likely to reflect true feelings as opposed to censored verbal interpretations generated by the CIA.

A convincing case has been made by Pelletier showing how modern humans are always under stress. The sympathetic nervous system provides the first response to stress, the "fight or flight" options. However, neither of these is a viable alternative for most modern stressors; we cannot attack or flee from an irritating boss, traffic jam or stack of bills. Without discharge of the programmed response, "a prolonged and unabated stress response" by the sympathetic nervous system ensues, leading eventually to exhaustion or to an explosive, hysterical response such as violence and addiction to stress and intensity. Pelletier adds a provocative thought on this a few pages later:

> It is possible that twentieth century man has designed a social and economic structure which is antipathetic to his health and psychological well-being. If this is so, can an evolutionary change help us adapt in a new version of survival of the fittest? Will the social system regulate itself when it becomes evident that its psychological complexity is affecting its members negatively? Or will man take it upon himself to scale down the proliferation of technological progress and concentrate upon a more inner-directed quest to preserve his mental and physical equilibrium?[62]

The idea of a chronically stressful life has many implications in medicine, psychology, sociology, economics and politics. It accounts for the dramatic effect of the sympathetic balance contacts in Polarity Therapy bodywork, and the popularity of mood-altering intoxicants and medications, which allow the system temporary (the problem is not being addressed) rest from chronic stress.

–JC

---

[62] Pelletier, Kenneth. *Mind as Healer, Mind as Slayer.* Pages 69 and 82.

5. How Involution and Evolution Create the Emotions

The mind, feelings and body are linked in a chain of cause and effect, constantly cycling from the subtle to the dense, from the mind to the body, and back. As we have discussed, the many manifestations of this cycle are reflections of the larger cosmic cycle of involution and evolution, by which a soul travels into creation and ultimately returns to its Source.

Motor and Sensory

Stone used the words "motor" and "sensory" to describe these two sides. The motor function is the movement from blueprint through motivation into materialization. The sensory function is the movement from materialization through feelings back to blueprint.

The feedback from the sensory function is the only way for the motor function to know if its efforts are successful. Without the moon, the sun cannot know itself. If the feedback is painful, the next impulse of the motor current will be adapted to seek a more successful result.

For a simple example, analyze the act of eating. The blueprint (mind) is pre-programmed to create actions to satisfy the need. Based on sensory input, edible material is perceived. A motor impulse is generated, causing the hand to reach out to satisfy the need. A sensory return message then tells whether the motor action was successful. If the food was too hot, the sensory message protects the person from being burned. The next motor response will be adapted appropriately.

The situation is similar, but more complex, for emotional issues. All children are programmed at birth with basic etheric needs, which are real and valid for all children. The motor currents will initiate action to fulfill those needs, and the sensory currents will guide adaptation by giving feedback on those actions.

Using the Polarity model of the Five Elements, the basic emotional necessities are the needs for security (Earth), belonging (Water), warmth (Fire), hope (Air), and expression (Ether). All of these are given and received to varying degrees through parental love for the child. Pia Mellody has given a very useful five innate qualities of the child which fit nicely: the child is (and has a right to be) vulnerable (Earth), dependent (Water), imperfect (Fire), immature (Air) and valuable (Ether).[63]

The young child spontaneously initiates motor activity to have these needs met, manifesting the five innate qualities as it does. The nature of these actions is a function of the child's blueprint, which combines traits from that family with traits common to all others of that sex.

Immediately after conception, even before birth, sensory messages begin to flow to the child. The game has begun for this lifetime. Motor actions go out, sensory feedback comes back in a continuous loop of action and reaction.

Search for Love

In the child's search for love in the five elemental categories, inevitable frustrations and traumas occur. Perhaps the parents do not feel secure themselves, so the sensory feedback indicates danger. Perhaps the child's innate qualities are denied, due to parental inability to function in a mature way.

Feedback alerts the new mind to the problem. New motor actions attempt to resolve the problem, or adapt in such a way as to extract a garbled, limited form of love, making the best of the situation.

Adapted strategies soon become habits, for unpredictability is more stressful than limited love. Strategies

---

[63] Mellody, Pia. *Facing Codependence.* p. 113.

which lead to love set the stage for successful emotional navigation later in life. Adapted strategies which are unsuccessful in gaining love set the stage for lives of pain. Mellody specifically identifies the types of adaptation which result from frustration of each of the five original motives, complete with the adult dysfunctional symptoms that inevitably result. The symptoms are problems with: boundaries (Earth); needs (Water); knowing and expressing one's reality (Fire); moderation (Air); self-esteem (Ether).

Once the adaptation is established, new situations are not analyzed on their own merits, but rather from the skewed perspective of a faulty blueprint. Our judgement does not mature past this point in time of childhood emotional injury.

Only by changing the blueprint, a difficult task later in life, can these patterns of pain be transformed. Accessing and reprograming these subconscious blueprint-level mental patterns is the goal of emotional therapy.

Energy Blocks

Adaptation also interrupts the cycle of involution and evolution. In the presence of pain, we block the reception of sensory feedback or withhold the expression of motor action. This can occur at four points in the cycle: the involutionary side can withhold action or ignore feedback, while the evolutionary side can block the receiving of action or distort the feedback. These problems are locked physically in the body as energy blocks.

The greatest challenge in healing the emotions is overcoming the momentum of habitual patterns. As part of pain management, we deny its presence. Because we are immersed in dysfunctional patterns, we cannot see them. Thus the first priority is to become aware of how we are feeling, and accept the reality of those feelings. This is the road to the blueprint, from which lasting changes can be made.

Thus the therapeutic process is parallel to the larger "Journey of the Soul" process. Just as the soul eventually awakens to its plight of separation from its source, the healing of emotional problems requires an awakening to their presence. From the pain of dysfunctional family histories we become motivated to start the quest for self-understanding, and ultimately for God understanding.

-JC

6. Integrating Chinese and Polarity Systems

The question is sometimes asked, how the Chinese energy anatomy and therapy model fits with the Polarity model. The two systems seem to be different in some respects, although the underlying theories are generally quite similar. They are thought to share a common origin in very ancient times, although the history is not known.

The success of acupuncture is a testament to the insight of ancient Chinese practitioners, and an indigestible thought for the Newtonian western medical model. Kinesiology deserves appreciation for advancing this ancient wisdom into the modern scene, and today's Polarity practitioner can benefit greatly from information presented in the many Kinesiology systems.

How can we compare the two ancient systems theoretically? Why does acupuncture work, from a Polarity perspective? Stone considered the systems identical:

> ...the old Ayurvedic Medicine and Acupuncture ascribed three modes of motion to energy in the three dimensions of space, and called them the three "Gunas" - "Satva" the neuter, "Rajas" the positive, and "Tamas" the negative mode of motion. The Chinese called them the "Qi" (neuter), the "Yang" (positive) and the "Yin" (negative) poles of action. These became the Air, Fire and Water [Principles] of the Hermetic philosophers, who obtained this information from the Orient.

> ...Acupuncture classifies all organs as either positive or negative, with many qualifications and points of contact for inserting the gold (positive) needle for disbursing and distributing excess energy; or the negative pole, the silver needle, for toning areas as specific spots. The balancing of the two extremes made a blend in which the neuter "Qi" energy could

flow again and link these poles to the Life Current of the Universal Essence, by tuning in; even as male and female are united in the child, the ever-becoming Youth of Life.

Acupuncture balances the two currents in their function and polarity with each other by means of needles, so they will flow in and out of the form freely in normal action and expression, called Health or Well-being. When there is no obstruction to the current energy flow, there is no pain or stagnation in the circulation.

WHAT THE NEEDLES CAN DO, THE HANDS CAN DO BETTER, with a battery of consciousness behind them plus intelligence for direction of currents. The right hand is the positive sun action, radiating, disbursing, outgoing golden energy. The left hand is the negative cooling moon energy, toning, soothing and inhibiting or concentrating the current for sedimentation and use. (Stone, *Polarity Therapy Vol. 2.* p. 208)

While this gives a general sense of similarity, several points of interest remain. How do the acupuncture meridians (the Chinese system energy current mappings) make sense from a Polarity perspective? A possible answer is given in Gerber's *Vibrational Medicine*.[64] This summarizes research (by Kim Bong Han of Korea and Pierre de Vernejoul of France) tracking the movement of radioactive isotopes injected into acupuncture points.

The patterns which emerge indicate the existence of a microductal system which parallels but precedes (is created earlier in the embryo) the formation of vascular and lymphatic ductal systems. This system seems to lay out energy pathways to shape the creation of tissues, and to be closely linked with autonomic nervous system function.

[64] Gerber, Richard. *Vibrational Medicine.* p. 122.

In Polarity terminology, these functions (creation of tissues and autonomic nervous system) are theoretically the action of the Yang Principle, the involutionary side of the energy equation. Thus stimulation of acupuncture meridians with needles, heat or touch may be energy balancing which is tracking the Yang Principle.

A complementary hypothesis can be made about the other great arm of Chinese medicine, herbalism, being a treatment based on the Yin energy Principle. In Polarity bodywork, the Yang Principle is the basis for many techniques, especially contacts involving the Interlaced Triangles, umbilicus, "Path of Fire," back and diaphragm.

Another topic of interest here is the relationship of the Chinese Five Elements to the Polarity Five Elements.

Are these terms referring to the same phenomena, and how do they match up? Kaptchuk's *The Web That Has No Weaver: Understanding Chinese Medicine* offers an explanation.

First, the Chinese Five Elements are properly translated as "Five Phases."

> The Theory of the Five Phases is an attempt to classify phenomena in terms of five quintessential processes, represented by the emblems Wood, Fire, Earth, Metal and Water... The Five Phases are not in any way matter.[65]

These phases correspond to the natural cycle of growth and decay exemplified in the seasons. From this general beginning based on Yang (Spring and Summer), Yin (Fall and Winter) and Qi (Transition), Kaptchuk describes how the Five Phases idea became rigid, losing some of its usefulness in modern Chinese medicine. Interpretations have varied from age to age and practitioner to practitioner.

To the degree that equivalents can be drawn to Polarity, the following seems to apply for Elemental correspondences:

---

[65] Kaptchuk, Ted. *The Web That Has No Weaver.* p. 199 and p. 343.

Polarity	Chinese
Ether	Earth
Air	Wood
Fire	Fire
Water	Metal
Earth	Water

The sequential unfolding of the Chinese Five Phases is very similar to the sequential densities of the Polarity Five Elements. However, there are also differences: for example, the Chinese Five Phases are identified with organs and functions which do not always seem to fit the corresponding Polarity descriptions. For this reason, the equation of the two systems does not seem to hold up completely. The whole context in which these originated and are applied is so different that it does not seem valuable to pursue the equation too deeply. Rather, each system of Elements should be appreciated on its own merits.

If anything, the interest in comparison is better focused on the Chinese Qi/Yang/Yin and Polarity Satva/Rajas/Tamas Principles, which are the cores of both systems and virtually identical, as we saw in the passage from Stone. As Kaptchuk describes the resemblance in the same pages:

> Similarities to the Chinese model are found even in non-bipolar systems, such as the Hindu Ayurvedic system. For example, Pitha [Rajasic Principle]... resembles China's Yang; Vata [the Satvic Principle]... resembles China's Qi, and Kapha [the Tamasic Principle] very much resembles China's Yin... When I worked in an Ayurvedic Hospital in India years ago, I found that my Chinese medical background enabled me in a short time to predict the categories that Ayurvedic physicians would use to describe their patients.

-JC

7. Yin and Yang, Gender and the Life Lesson

The Polarity model gives a useful perspective on the meaning of gender. Why is one person a man (and thus inevitably challenged biologically by Yang experience, in addition to Yin experience which will arise to varying degrees), and another a woman (and thus inevitably challenged biologically by Yin experience, in addition to Yang experience which will arise to varying degrees)? Is this accidental? Such questions penetrate to the deepest levels of human inquiry, to the Journey of the Soul subject matter that Stone considered the essence of Polarity Therapy. Polarity Therapy is exceptional in its ability to venture into this realm of existential philosophy.

Stone explains human life as a quest for knowledge and experience. The fact of gender fits in with this quest. A student returning to college after vacation, does not choose courses that are already known, but rather those with new challenges.

Similarly, the soul seeks fields of action in experience which represent new challenge. In traditional Japanese folklore, it is said that the sex of the child is a function of the challenge of the parents. A child will be born into a male body if the progress of the soul requires Yang lessons (possibly having dealt previously and successfully with Yin challenges), and the child will be born to parents who, at that time, are creating a field of action in which the appropriate Yang challenges will be certain to manifest.

Thus the fact of gender is a matter to be appreciated, not minimized. This perspective is confirmed by one of Stone's esoteric sources, *The Emerald Tablet of Hermes,* (Stone, *Polarity Therapy Vol. 2.* Book 6, p. 27) which places the meaning of gender as one of its six core concepts. All experience, from smallest to largest dimension, follows from the fundamental event of gender identity. The qualities of sperm and egg manifest throughout our experience, bringing us the lessons of life.

The attraction and repulsion of Yang and Yin is an expression of the essential nature of energy, culminating in intercourse and conception and providing the family matrix for the raising of children. The magnetic emotional force of sexual attraction and the miraculous dynamics of conception are perhaps the most remarkable demonstrations of the workings of energy in human experience.

It is a measure of the grand illusion of life that so much controversy has arisen on issues of sexual identity and role. Stone emphasized that both sexes are on the same spiritual path:

> WOMEN, AS WELL AS MEN, have the same right
> and footing in both processes [involution and evolu-
> tion]. (Stone, *Polarity Therapy Vol. 1.* Book 1, p. 40)

Deeper issues await us: we can see this body, male or female, as a meaningful temporary vehicle for the learning of certain lessons, and go on to the search for understanding of what our individual lessons are and how we can successfully learn them.

> This gross body, I cannot be. Why? I am seeing it. It
> is an object for my sight. I am the seer. It is separate
> and I am separate. (Stone, *Polarity Therapy Vol. 2.* Book 6,
> p. 28)

-JC

8. The Three Principles of Polarity and Three Dimensions of Edu-K

We can understand energy systems easier by looking at the body as an energetic three dimensional figure moving through time and space. These three dimensions of height, width and depth can be analyzed in terms of posture, movement and energy circuits. This study is central to both Polarity Therapy and to Edu-K, the effective brain-integration therapy developed by Paul Dennison.

Back-Front

This first dimension or direction of action has three possibilities: moving out or expanding, moving in or contracting, and stillness or maintaining sameness. As we move forward, we go out to meet situations and people. As we move back, we are more within ourselves and less accessible to outside influences. We may use the inward movement to digest and process experience. In the middle or neutral space we have the opportunity to move in or out, and take in or give out.

When we are functioning optimally, all these modes are accessible to us and we can choose whichever is appropriate at any given moment. Our posture, both in general and at each moment, reflects our status of outward and inward, back and forward. This dimension also reflects the communication between the back and front brains, connecting the past with the present, the visual experience with expression.

In the Dennisons' Educational Kinesiology, this understanding of the back/front dimension is called 'Focus' and has to do with our ability to focus on things outside ourselves while maintaining our own integrity. We might evaluate our ability to focus by seeing whether we can look at a book, TV show or another person and learn from them while keeping ourselves in perspective. When our energies are out of balance in this dimension, we may be over- or under-focused, "too out" or "too in."

In a state of over-focus we deplete ourselves and lose our sense of self as we become engrossed in something outside ourselves. Posturally, this would appear as a forward head and stooped shoulders. In a state of under-focus, we are unable to focus on things because we are so much inside ourselves that it is too much of a strain to allow the energy to go out. Posturally, we would see this in a holding back stance. This dimension has to do with comprehension or understanding. Understanding comes from the ability to interact with something outside ourselves and bring it within in a meaningful and balanced context.

This dimension may be compared to the Yang Principle in Polarity, in which concentric spirals radiate outward from the umbilical or solar plexus area. This has to do with the ability to produce heat and warmth and to put our fiery creativity into expression in interaction with other people and situations. It also relates to our ability to take in and digest experience. The eyes are very much part of the fire. We feel that fire when someone else's anger or warmth is directed toward us through their eyes. We use the fire of the eyes to take in and digest visual cues and written words. This relates to our ability to focus, to allow that fire of the eyes to look outside and in.

Top-Bottom

In the second dimension, we look at the energies that move up and down. As these energies flow, it is a link between our foundation and our manifestation, our reflex and cognition, our denser and finer energies, between the upper and lower centers of the brain. We constantly balance higher aspirations and practical limitation. The term "grounded" has frequently been used to describe this relationship: ungrounded meaning disassociation from feelings or unrealistic attitudes, over-grounded meaning lacking a higher vision of potential achievement.

In the Dennisons' work, this dimension is called "Centering" and the word that is associated with it is "organization." This dimension reflects how the body organizes its flow through life and whether events throw us off center or we maintain our center.

In Stone's work, these longitudinal currents relate to the Yin Principle. As the currents flow downward into the denser areas of the body, they may crystallize and be blocked in their return upward. In the drawing of the energy man, these currents are represented by the lines moving through the fingers and toes. These are similar in flow to the longitudinal nature of acupuncture meridians.

Left-Right

The third dimension is left to right or side to side. This dimension reflects the communication between the two sides of the brain hemispheres, Yin and Yang, male and female, receptive and outgoing, analytic and feeling. It deals with fine, quickly-moving energy, as quick as the changing of our minds.

In Educational Kinesiology this dimension is named "Laterality" and deals with the idea of "communication." This dimension represents our ability to cross the midline of vision, hearing, thought, etc. and use the information of both sides to respond in an integrated or whole brain fashion. This is especially important for reading and writing skills. People commonly experience stress and a lack of integration for crossing the midline and those with severe difficulties are often diagnosed as dyslexic. Through the Dennisons' pioneering work with integration of the brain hemispheres, much progress has been made in working with dyslexia.

In Polarity Therapy, this is the Satvic (Satva means truth in Sanskrit) or Neutral Principle. It is represented by the side-to-side current spinning transversely about the body.

Dimensions and Exercises

In working with exercise and balance, we approach all three dimensions or principles in the type of movement we do and the type of touch we use.

The back-front dimension or fiery Rajas/Yang principle is stimulated by rocking movements and fiery sounds. The Edu-K "focus aspect" as seen in postural cues is released by all Brain Gym lengthening exercises which release the tendon guard reflex holding pattern and allow the body to once again participate with the outer and inner worlds.

The up-down Tamas or Yin currents are affected in Polarity by bringing them closely together to build on each other and by deep, releasing touch, especially on the feet. These currents are also balanced with movements and contacts that connect longitudinal lines and meridians. In Edu-K, all Button contacts accomplish this "Centering" system by affecting meridian flow. Proper hydration is important here. Without the appropriate amount of water for ionization and chemical processing, the electrochemistry cannot function correctly.

The side-to-side Satva or Neutral currents are balanced in Polarity by gentle touch and side to side movement, followed by pauses which bring stillness balance to the middle. In Edu-K the issue of "Crossing the midline" is often addressed by exercises which take the mind and body from one side to the other using the figure eight shape.

We sometimes choose exercises by using the image of the three dimensions to get a feel for our current state. The following chart gives an understanding of emotional/mental states relating each dimension and a menu of appropriate exercises for balancing each. Wonderful self-help sessions can be developed based on this approach.

Symptoms & Menus for Brain Integration

Dimension	Switched Off	Switched On	Menu
Left-Right Laterality Satva Communication	Struggling, polarized, oppositional, win-lose, unable to communicate, feelings and thoughts in conflict, words and feeling not integrated, inner and outer don't match, indulgent, uncoordinated, feeling blocked	Effortless Effort, both sides, mental flexibility, access to alternatives, win-win, inner communication, outer communication, inner harmony, consistency between inner and outer, coordination	<u>Polarity:</u> Scissors kicks, Side to side and Pierre Ha Breath, Sensory balance **Brain Gym:** Cross crawl, Lazy 8s, Belly breathing, Sacral Rock, Shoulder Shrug Neck Rolls, Dennison Laterality Repatterning
Bottom- Top Centering Tamas Organization	Off center, pushover, stubborn, frozen, stuck, scattered, shattered, unable to manifest ideals in a grounded way, easily thrown off, disorganized	Centered, stable, sense of integrity, balance, organization, stability with movement, flexibility with grounding, ideals manifest in daily life	<u>Polarity:</u> Pyramid, squat, rowing, diaphragm press **Brain Gym:** Buttons series: Brain, Earth, Balance, Space; Thinking cap
Back-Front Focus Rajas Participation	Pulled back, withdrawn, dependent, lost in tasks or other people, putting others ahead of self, over- or under-focused, can't remember or integrate info, needy, neglecting self	Participating, good sense of self, understanding, memory comprehension, giving and receiving, expressive, ability to be with self and other, balanced perspective	<u>Polarity:</u> Motor balance, Sciatic Ha, Lion Roar, Wise Man of Old, Humming, Pyramid, Squat, Diaphragm press **Brain Gym:** Owl, Foot flex, Arm activation, Hamstring & Psoas lengthening
Deepening Attitudes Peace	Agitated, confused, unclear, physical discomfort, reactive, energy drain, upset, depressed, overwhelmed	Calm, peaceful, clarity, feeling good, capable, compassionate, energetic	<u>Polarity:</u> Sensory balance, Five-pointed star **Brain Gym:** Cook's Hookups, Positive points

-MLM

9. What is Stress?

Stress is commonly considered one of the great maladies of modern society. We have created lifestyles and environments that constantly stress our entire being. Ancient stresses of the struggle for survival have been replaced with more complex pressures of time, money and a thousand other tensions.

Hans Selye, author and pioneer stress researcher, found stress difficult to describe. His simple definition was, "the non-specific response of the body to any demand made upon it." The demand, called a "stressor," is neither negative nor positive but simply requires a response. Even the most delightful changes in our lives can be stressful for us. In this age of rapid growth and change, we are continually challenged to adapt with equanimity and balance. Many of our stressors come from our need for stimulation and growth; and we would not do without them, for they enliven and challenge us. Others we need to change, for they will hurt us in the long run. Energy Exercises help release tension, but we must remember that the ability to discriminate between positive and negative stressors, and to seek ways to reduce negative influences precedes exercise as a stress management strategy.

As we meet daily stresses, many of us have chosen to ignore or over-ride the body's natural feedback to us. The use of alcohol, caffeine, nicotine, painkillers and other drugs is symptomatic of the stresses of our modern lifestyle and our difficulty in managing them.

One of the themes of this book, and of Polarity Therapy, is personal responsibility. These are methods to take stresses in our lives and process them, to use our personal energy to enliven and grow rather than contract and suffer.

Where do stresses affect our bodies? It can be anywhere. There are many conditions currently considered to be stress related: heart disease, stroke, asthma, ulcers, migraine headaches, colitis, rheumatoid arthritis, depression, etc. All people are more prone to disease when they have been under stress, so we could consider all disease to be stress-related. When we experience stress, we might feel neck and shoulder tension, back aches, headaches, fatigue, over-reactivity, tightness in the chest, depression, poor concentration and/or chronic anxiety.

The body responds to stress by calling in the guard. The initial response is called the "alarm reaction" or "fight or flight response". The sympathetic nervous system activates and the body sets off hormonal activities which send messages to get ready for quick action. Blood pressure, heart rate, respiration, sweat and muscle tension increase while non-essential processes related to the digestive, urinary and reproductive systems are cut back. Though the breathing rate increases, the breath itself becomes shallower and we feel the state of stress in our body as the tension and shallowness of breath. We may also experience heart palpitation, weakness, knots in the stomach or other symptoms. Ideally, we respond in some way that ends the stress. Then we can relax and allow our body to re-adjust.

In some cases however, the stress persists and a second stage of response occurs called the resistance reaction. This allows the body to continue its readied state after the initial alarm reaction has dissipated. The blood chemistry returns to nearly normal, but the blood pressure remains high due to the blood volume increase from water retention. In most problems, this is the highest stage of stress response we reach before we return to normal.

However when the stress persists and this stage is not successful, the body will move to the stage of exhaustion. Cells become depleted as they use more and more potassium. They function less effectively and finally start to die. A strong long-term resistance reaction wears on the body, particularly the heart, blood vessels and adrenal cortex. The body may not be able to meet the heavy demands or may suddenly fail with the strain. Our ability to handle stressors is largely determined by our general health and the baseline from which we operate.

Obviously we wish to prevent this exhaustion. We cannot necessarily change the factors creating stress, but we can change our responses to them, and we can create a foundation level of vitality and general health that can meet the stresses we are exposed to.

Different people carry their stresses differently. We all tend to have a vulnerable spot where we feel things first as our body begins to feel pressure. We can use our own connection with the feeling of discomfort in this area as an automatic alarm system telling us to take a stress release break. This feedback function is a natural value of (and reason for) pain.

We tend to have certain common tightening responses to stress. The tendon guard reflex is our natural primitive defense. You can picture this when you imagine a lizard freezing in place when startled. In our bodies, we similarly freeze and lock the back. The knees become rigid and we tighten up the underside of the foot, the muscles in the back of the calves and thighs and up the spine when we feel threatened. In many activities, we work with the muscles involved in this reflex and help them to release their tension.

- MLM

10. Exercises in a Chair

Exercise is for everyone. Youthful people in good health can easily do the exercises in this book, but the unwell, overweight and elderly can have difficulty. Don't be discouraged! If the obstacles are greater (and the beginning will be the hardest), the potential for change is also greater. There is always a way to exercise.

This list is for people of limited exercise capability. All these can be done while seated in a chair, with little effort.

Breathing is emphasized even more than usual. With each position take time to breathe deeply and fully, really emphasizing the exhale. This does not mean any form of hyperventilation, but rather deep and relaxed breathing with plenty of rest as needed.

These exercises are listed in a series which can be done in sequence, omitting any which are too difficult or time consuming. This sequence is not fixed: experiment with other orders or do just the favorite or most appropriate postures.

11. Exercises for Pregnancy

This list gives exercises which are particularly valuable during pregnancy. Generally, only a few of the exercises in this book are contraindicated for pregnancy. As a rule, avoid exercises which are painful (such as deep pressure on the feet or calves) or which require extreme exertion (such as Rowing with great resistance and Woodchopper). The Up and Down Ha Breath should not be done rapidly or forcefully.

Attitudes are emphasized during pregnancy. We advocate a peaceful, low pressure lifestyle during this time especially. We believe that the baby "sees" and "hears" everything that happens while in the womb. Security is a top priority. Talking to the baby (make him or her feel wanted), enjoying soft music and natural scenery, and optimistic, positive thoughts are valuable during this time.

Exercise	Page
Squat	51
Pyramid	48
Rocking Perineal	57
Sacral Rock	59
Cliffhanger	19
Diaphragm exercises (be gentle!)	28
Buttons series	72
Cook's Hook Ups	67
Positive Points	75
Seated Scissors Kick	56
Humming	84

In addition, the following are useful exercises for pregnancy. These are well-known in birth classes.

• **Pelvic Tuck:** On all fours, alternately flex and release the pelvis.
• **Partial Inversion:** Lying head down on a slanted surface relieves gravity pressure.
• **Kegels:** Tighten and relax internal muscles of the pelvic floor.

Glossary of Terms

Activation: An exercise technique which uses muscle pressure against light resistance to relax the muscle. Similar to isometric exercise, but more gentle and for relaxation more than strength building.

Air Element: The second element and level of materialization, the gases. Centered in the chest.

Ayurveda: The traditional medicine of northern India, one of the primary sources for Polarity Therapy.

Bi-Polar Current: The movement of the Yin Principle, from top to bottom and back. Also called Long-line or Longitudinal current.

Bioenergetics: A therapeutic system created by Alexander Lowen.

Breathing: An exercise technique in which the breath is consciously controlled and observed.

Centrifugal treatment: In bodywork, treatment from the inside-out and/or the top-down, emphasizing involutionary function.

Centripetal treatment: In bodywork, treatment from the outside-in and/or the bottom-up, emphasizing evolutionary function.

Craniosacral Therapy: A therapeutic system indirectly derived from Osteopathic Medicine. It is based on understanding the movements, qualities, roles and relationships of cranium, spinal system and sacrum.

Diaphragm: The large dome-shaped muscle in the solar plexus.

Differentiation: An exercise technique in which the movements of muscles are isolated from habitual groups, for relaxation and self-discovery.

Earth Element: The fifth element and level of materialization. Centered in the pelvic floor.

Elements, Five: See Five Elements

Energy: A general term for the primal force which creates, sustains and destroys all phenomena.

Energy Balancing: A term for working with subtle fields and pathways to restore the natural flow of current in the body.

Ether Element: The subtlest level of materialization, the space in which the lower four elements are created. A reflection of the Neutral Principle. Centered at the throat.

Fire Element: The third level element and level of materialization, heat. Centered in the solar plexus.

Five Elements: The second (after the Three Principles) level of differentiation applied to phenomena, referring to the increasing density of manifestation as spirit moves into matter. They can be thought of as the space, gas, heat, liquids and solids of all existence.

Five Pointed Star: The geometric pattern of the Yin Principle.

Hallucis tendon: A tendon which attaches the big toe to the lower leg, used in energy balancing bodywork. Its main access point is on the inside of the ankle.

Interlaced Triangles: The geometric pattern of the Yang Principle.

Kinesiology: A natural biofeedback system using muscles as indicators of underlying energy movement. Systems using kinesiology include Touch for Health, Edu-K, Hyperton-x, PHP (Professional Health Provider) and One Brain.

Lengthening: An exercise technique in which the range of potential motion of a muscle is increased.

Longitudinal Current: The movement of the Yin Principle, from top to bottom and back. Also called Long-line or Bi-polar current.

Martial Arts: A general term for the physical disciplines of the far East, including T'ai Ch'i and others. These were based on Polarity ideas and had the goals of self-understanding and living in harmony with nature.

Meridians: Energy current circuits in Chinese acupuncture, thought to trace the pathway of the Yang Principle.

Motor: The functions of the Yang Principle

Pannetier, Pierre: (1914-1984) One of Stone's best known Polarity Therapy students and a successful teacher of Polarity in America.

Polarity: The idea of two interdependent forces. It is the foundation of several energy-based health systems, Eastern philosophy and modern physical science.

Prana: A Sanskrit term for the subtle life force of energy which rides on the air.

Pressure: An exercise technique involving touch, for energy balancing, tissue release or easing tension.

Principles, Three: See Three Principles.

Rajas: A Sanskrit term for the positive, Yang Principle.

Reflexology: The concept that different parts of the body are linked by invisible connections, being reflections of each other.

Satva: Sanskrit term for the Neutral Principle.

Sensory: The functions of the Yin Principle.

Six Pointed Star: See Interlaced Triangles, which is the preferred term.

Stillpoint: In Craniosacral Therapy, a healing moment when the body relaxes and self-adjusts. The term refers specifically to a pause in the cranial pulsation or rhythm.

Tamas: A Sanskrit term for the negative, Yin Principle.

Three Principles: The first and most basic differentiation applied to primal Energy. They can be thought of as the beginning, the middle and the end of any event, or as going out, coming back and stillness. See the table on page 271.

Transverse Current: The movement of the Neutral Principle, from side-to-side in a spiral shape.

Umbilical Current: The movement of the Yang Principle, a spiral radiating out from the Umbilicus. Also called the Spiral current.

Water Element: The fourth element and level of materialization, liquids. Centered in the pelvis.

Wu-Wei: Literally, "effortless effort" of east Asian physical discipline systems.

Yang: The Chinese term for the active, involutionary side of any manifestation of energy.

Yin: The Chinese term for the reactive, evolutionary side of any manifestation of energy.

Yoga: Literally, Union. Ancient systems of self-discipline and self realization from India, and a source for these exercises. Hatha Yoga refers to Yang (Ha, Sun) and Yin (Sun and Moon) interdependence.

Terminology Guide to the Three Principles

Field	Yang	Yin	Neutral
Electrical charge	+, Heating	-, Cooling	0, Neutral, reversing
Direction	Centrifugal	Centripetal	Reversal, stillness
Ayurveda	Pitta, Pingala	Kapha, Ida	Vata, Sushumna
Dimension	Back-Front	Bottom-Top	Side to side
Body Function	Arteries, Motor Nerves, Inhale, Flexion	Veins, Sensory Nerves, Exhale, Extension	Heart & Capillaries, CNS, Reversal, Joints
Embryonic	Ectoderm	Endoderm	Mesoderm
Current flow	Steady rhythmic, action	Cyclic, changing, reaction	Stillness, reversal
Gender	Male, sperm	Female, egg	Consciousness
Phases	Cardinal	Mutable	Fixed
Time	Beginning, Summer	Ending, winter	Middle, Solstice, Equinox
Bodywork	Stimulating	Deep tissue	Balancing
Religious	Father, Vishnu, Creator	Son, Shiva, Destroyer	Holy Ghost, Brahma, Sustainer
Archetypes	Benevolent King or Father	Nurturing Queen or Mother	Wise Counselor
Unbalanced archetypes	Tyrant, Wimp	Critic, Doormat	
Lifestyle protection	Avoid Intoxicants	Avoid Promiscuity	Vegetarian diet
Perspective	Objective Observer	Subjective Participant	Access to both
Attitude	Dispassionate	Impassioned	Compassionate
Processing center	Brain	Pelvis	Heart

Terminology Guide to the Five Elements

Field	Ether	Air	Fire	Water	Earth
Chakra	Throat, *Vishuda*	Chest, *Anahata*	Solar Plexus, *Manipura*	Pelvis, *Savadhistana*	Pelvic Floor, *Muladhara*
Emotions	Grief/Joy, Expression, Choice	Greed/ Generosity, Hope	Anger/Will Power, being Determined	Lust/ Discipline, Attachment	Fear/ Courage, Grounding
Primary Quality	Self-esteem	Moderation	Self-knowledge, being realistic	Self-care	Self protection
Color	Blue	Green	Yellow	Orange	Red
Body	Throat, thyroid	Chest, Heart/ Lungs	Solar Plexus, digestion	Pelvis, Reproductive	Bones
Astrological Triads and body areas	(No astrological sign) Joints, diaphragms	Gemini (shoulders), Libra (Kidneys), Aquarius (ankles	Aries (head), Leo, Solar plexus), Sagittarius (thighs)	Cancer (breast), Scorpio (genitals), Pisces (feet)	Taurus (neck), Virgo (intestines), Capricorn (knees)
Vocation	Spirituality, art	Education, commercial art	Industry, commerce, sports	Nurturing, caregiving, education	Security, military
Verbal probe	"I feel____"	"I want ____"	"I will ____"	"I need ____"	"I fear ____"
Sense	Sound	Touch	Sight	Taste	Smell
Fingers & Toes	Thumb, big toe	Pointer, 2nd toe	Middle, 3rd toe	Ring, 4th toe	Littlest finger & toe
Endocrine	Thyroid	Thymus	Pancreas	Sex organs	Adrenals
Foods	Aesthetics, socializing & pacing	Tree-level fruits & nuts	Waist level grains	Knee Level veggies & greens	Ground level, root crops
Excess	Ungrounded	Speed, Greed	Anxious, domineering	Poor boundaries	Fear/ Courage, Grounding
Face	Expression	Eyebrows, cheeks	Diaphragm line, nose	Lips, mouth	Chin, jaw

Bibliography

Notes for the Revised Edition, 2017. This Bibliography was created in 1990 and is a good snapshot of resources available at that time. Of course, in subsequent years many new resources have appeared.

For Polarity Therapy, these are more recent books with updated bibliographies:

Chitty, John. *Dancing with Yin and Yang: Ancient Wisdom, Modern Psychotherapy and Randolph Stone's Polarity Therapy.* Polarity Press, Boulder CO, 2013.

Chitty, John. *Working with Babies: A Five-Step Therapy Method for Babies and Their Families.* Polarity Press, Boulder CO, 2016.

Arroyo, Stephen. *Astrology, Psychology and the Four Elements.* CRCS, Reno NV, 1975.

Bach-y-Rita, Eileen. *Feldenkrais at Home.* Cassette Series, Bach-y-Rita, Mill Valley CA, 1985.

Barhydt, Hamilton & Elizabeth. *Self-Help for Stress and Pain.* Loving Life, Auburn CA, 1989.

Beaulieu, John. *Music & Sound in the Healing Arts.* Station Hill Press, Barrytown NY, 1987.

Beaulieu, John. *Polarity Therapy Workbook.* BioSonic Enterprises, 1994.

Berkson, Devaki. *The Foot Book.* Barnes & Noble, New York NY, 1977.

Capra, Fritjof. *The Tao of Physics.* Shambala, Berkeley CA, 1975.

Chitty, Anna. *Man and Woman.* Video lecture, Murrieta Foundation, Murrieta CA, 1988.

Chopra, Deepak. *Quantum Healing.* Bantam, New York NY, 1989.

Cook, Wayne and Wanda, *Universal Truths.* Wanda Cook, Prescott AZ, 1988.

Cousins, Norman. *Head First.* Dutton, New York NY, 1989.

Dennison, Paul & Gail. *Brain Gym.* Edu-Kinesthetics, Glendale CA, 1986.

Dennison, Paul & Gail. *Edu-K for Kids.* Edu-Kinesthetics, Glendale CA, 1987.

Dennison, Paul & Gail. *Personalized Whole Brain Integration.* Edu-Kinesthetics, Glendale CA, 1985.

Dennison, Paul. *Switching On.* Edu-Kinesthetics, Glendale CA, 1981.

Diamond, John. *Your Body Doesn't Lie.* Warner, New York NY, 1979.

Dychtwald, Ken. *Bodymind.* Tarcher, Los Angeles CA, 1976.

Fast, Julius, *Body Language.* Pocket Books, New York NY, 1970.

Feldenkrais, Moshe. *Body & Mature Behavior.* International Universities Press, New York NY, 1973.

Feldenkrais, Moshe. *The Master Moves.* Meta, Cupertino CA, 1984.

Francis, John. *Polarity Self-Help Exercises.* APTA, Boston MA, 1989.

Gach, Michael. *Acu-Yoga.* Japan Publication, New York, NY, 1981.

Gerber, Richard, *Vibrational Medicine.* Bear & Co., Santa Fe NM, 1988.

Gordon, Richard. *Your Healing Hands.* Wingbow, Berkeley CA, 1984.

Govinda, Lama. *Foundations of Tibetan Mysticism.* Rider & Co., London England, 1960.

Gray, Robert. *The Colon Health Handbook.* Emerald, Reno NV, 1986.

Hay, Louise. *Heal Your Body.* Hay House, Santa Monica CA, 1984.

Horwitz, Tem. *Tai Chi Ch'uan.* Chicago Review Press, Chicago IL, 1976.

Jensen, Bernard. *Tissue Cleaning Through Bowel Management.* Jensen, Escondido CA, 1981.

Joudry, Patricia. *Sound Therapy for the Walkman.* Steele & Steele, St. Denis, Saskatchewan Canada, 1984.

Juhan, Deane. *Job's Body.* Station Hill Press, Barrytown NY, 1987.

Kaptchuk, Michael. *The Web That Has No Weaver*. Congdon & Weed, NY, 1983.

Keleman, Stanley. *Emotional Anatomy*. Center Press, Berkeley CA, 1985.

Kurtz, Ron & Prestera, Hector. *The Body Reveals*. Harper & Row, San Francisco CA, 1976.

Kurtz, Ron. *Hakomi Therapy*. Kurtz, Ashland OR, 1989.

Kushi, Michio. *The Book of Macrobiotics*. Japan Publications, Tokyo Japan and New York NY, 1977.

Lowen, Alexander. *Bioenergetics*. Penguin, New York NY, 1975.

Lowens, Alexander and Leslie. *The Way to Vibrant Health*. Harper, Colophon NY, 1977.

MacDougall, John and Mary. *The MacDougall Plan*. New Century, New York NY, 1983.

Mahoney, Frank. *Hyperton-X*. Hyperton-X, El Segundo CA, 1988.

Mellody, Pia. *Facing Codependence*. Harper & Row, San Francisco CA, 1989.

Muramoto, Naboru. *Healing Ourselves*. Avon, New York NY, 1973.

Pelletier, Kenneth. *Mind as Healer Mind as Slayer*. Delta/Dell, New York NY, 1977.

Robbins, John. *Diet for a New America*. Stillpoint, Walpole MA, 1987.

Robbins, Tony. *Unlimited Power*. Fawcett Columbine, New York NY, 1986.

Seidman, Maruti. *A Guide to Polarity Therapy*. Newcastle, Hollywood CA, 1986.

Siegel, Alan. *Polarity Therapy*. Prism Press, Dorset England, 1987.

Sills, Franklyn. *The Polarity Process*. Element Books, Dorset England, 1989.

Stokes, Daniel & Whiteside, Gordon. *Louder Than Words*. Three in One Concepts, Burbank CA, 1988.

Stokes, Daniel & Whiteside, Gordon. *One Brain*. Three in One Concepts, Burbank CA, 1987.

Stone, R. *Health Building*. CRCS, Sebastopol CA, 1986.

Stone, R. *Mystic Bible*. Radha Soami Satsang Beas, Delhi India, 1977.

Stone, R. *Polarity Therapy Vol. 1 and Vol. 2*. CRCS, Sebastopol CA, 1986 and 1987.

Thie, John. *Touch for Health*. DeVorss & Co, Marina del Rey CA, 1979.

Upledger, John. *CranioSacral Therapy I*. Eastland Press, Seattle WA, 1983.

Upledger, J. & Vredevoogd. *CranioSacral Therapy II*. Eastland Press, Seattle WA, 1987.

Welles, William. *The Hidden Crime of the Porcelain Throne*. Welles, San Diego CA, 1988. For information on Dr. Welles' products to assist with squatting: W. Welles, D.C., 4295 Gestner St., Ste 3A, San Diego, CA 92117. (619) 458-9210.

Wilhelm, Richard, translator. *The I Ching*. Princeton Univ. Press, Princeton NJ, 1971.

Young, Phil. *Polarity Therapy– where Energy Meets Structure and Function*. Masterworks International, 2017.

Zukav, Gary. *The Dancing Wu Li Masters*. Bantam, New York NY, 1980.

Index of References

The following is a list of all authors and references cited in this book. The works of Randolph Stone are excluded, being too numerous to meaningfully recount here.

References for Face Reading

Narayan S. Khalsa, Ph.D., has adopted an Ayurvedic perspective for comprehensive analysis of the face. His article "What's in a Face?" (Unpublished, 1985) cites the following references:

Bellak, L. and Baker, S.S., *Reading Faces*, Holt, Rinehart & Winston, New York NY, 1980.

Shen, P. and Wilson, J., *Face Fortunes: The Ancient Chinese Art of Feature Reading*, Perigree Books, New York NY, 1982.

Kushi, M., *Oriental Diagnosis: What Your Face*, Sunwheel Publications, London England, 1978.

Mar, T.T., *Face Reading*, Signet Books, New York NY, 1974.

Rinn, W.E., "The Neuropsychology of Facial Expression," *APA Journal*, 1984.

Stokes, G. and Whiteside, D. *Under the Code*, The Body/Mind Connection, 1979.

Trotter, R.J., "The Sign of Music Read in the Face," *Psychology Today*, March 1985, New York NY.

Ekman, P. and Friesen, W.V., *Unmasking the Face: A Guide to Recognizing Emotions from Facial Expressions*, Prentice Hall, Englewood Cliffs NJ, 1975.

Ekman, P. and Friesen, W.V., *Facial Action Coding System: Investigator's Guide*, Consulting Psychologists Press, Palo Alto CA, 1978.

Whiteside, D. and Stokes, G., "Louder than Words: The Structure Equals Function Connection," 1980.

Whiteside, R.L., *Facial Language*, Pocket Books, New York, 1975.

Young, L., *Secrets of the Face: The Chinese Art of Reading Character through Facial Structure and Features*, Little, Brown & Co., Boston, 1984.

Zajonc, R.B., "Emotion and Facial Efference: A Theory Reclaimed," *Science*, V. 228, 1984, pp. 15-21.

Index 1

Exercises Listed in Order of Appearance

Energy Exercises

Index 3
Illustrations and Diagrams
Listed in Order of Appearance

Energy Exercises

Also from Polarity Press

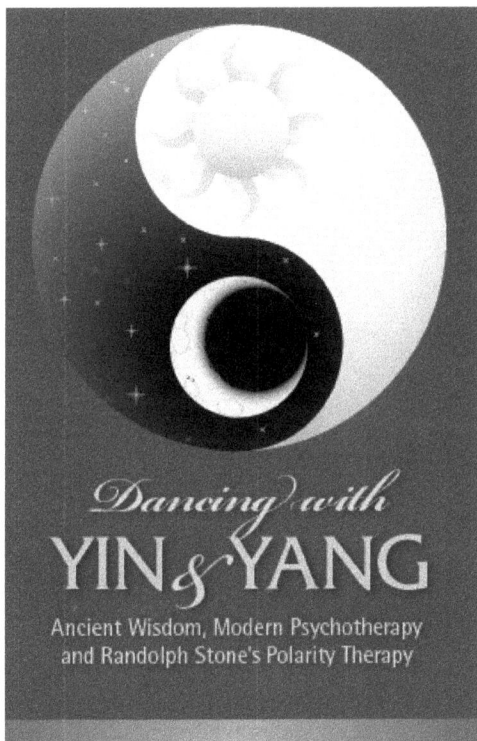

Dancing with Yin and Yang: Ancient Wisdom, Modern Psychotherapy and Randolph Stone's Polarity Therapy
by John Chitty
$25.95

The foundation book for study and practice of energy-based counseling and coaching. An entire paradigm of mental-emotional health care is offered, with numerous practical applications. This book includes a complete popular-style description of Polyvagal Theory, and a thorough explanation of Polarity's version of the Two-Chair method.

Working with Babies: A Five Part Therapy Method for Infants and their Families
By John Chitty
$19.95

This book combines Polarity Therapy, Biodynamic Craniosacral Therapy, prenatal psychology and trauma resolution to create a method for working with babies.

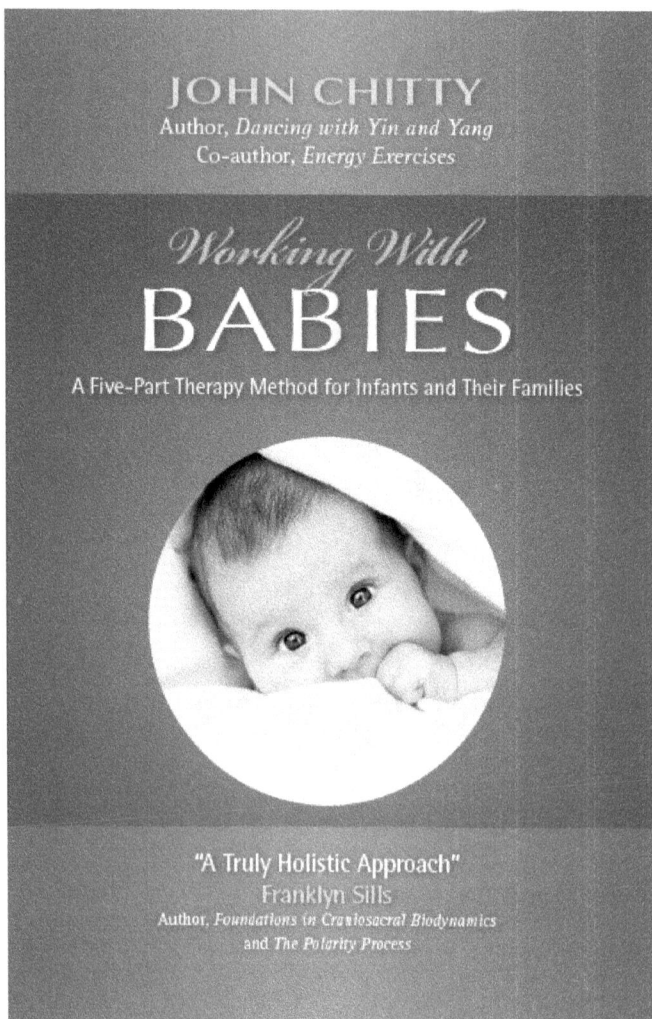

The Triune Autonomic Nervous System Wall Poster
by John Chitty
$24

This 18x24 color poster combines seven diagrams in one view to fully summarize the Polyvagal Theory. The diagrams are the same as those that illustrate Chapter 6 in *Dancing with Yin and Yang*. Additional commentary discusses implications of the theory.

Polarity Therapy Wall Charts
Art by Mark Allison, text by John Chitty
$7 each

These black and white 18x14 wall posters are based on some of Randolph Stone's most information-rich charts from *Polarity Therapy: The Complete Collected Works*.

WEAVING THE BODY

WIRELESS ANATOMY

ENERGY ZONES

5- AND 6-POINTED STARS

25 COMBINATIONS

www.ingramcontent.com/pod-product-compliance
Lightning Source LLC
Chambersburg PA
CBHW070740270326
41927CB00010B/2043